An Atlas of
HYPERTENSION

2nd Edition

THE ENCYCLOPEDIA OF VISUAL MEDICINE SERIES

An Atlas of
HYPERTENSION
2nd Edition

Peter F. Semple, MB, FRCP

Senior Lecturer and Consultant Physician
Department of Medicine and Therapeutics, Gardiner Institute
Western Infirmary, Glasgow, Scotland, UK

and

George B.M. Lindop, MB ChB, FRCP(Glasg), FRCPath

Senior Lecturer and Consultant in Histopathology
University Department of Pathology
Western Infirmary, Glasgow, Scotland, UK

Foreword by

John H. Laragh, MD

Hilda Altschul Master Professor of Medicine and Director, Cardiovascular Center
The New York Hospital–Cornell Medical Center
New York, NY, USA

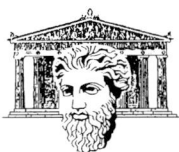

The Parthenon Publishing Group
International Publishers in Medicine, Science & Technology

NEW YORK   LONDON

Library of Congress Cataloging-in-Publication Data
Semple, Peter F.
        An atlas of hypertension / Peter F. Semple and George B.M. Lindop
: foreword by John H. Laragh. -- 2nd ed.
                p.   cm. -- (The Encyclopedia of Visual Medicine Series)
        Includes bibliographic references and index.
        ISBN 1-85070-949-1
        I. Hypertension--Diagnosis--Atlases. I. Lindop, George B.M.,
1945–   . II. Title. III. Series.
        [DNLM: I. Hypertension--diagnosis--atlases. 2. Diagnostic
Imaging--atlases. WG 17 S473a 1997]
RC685.H8S46 1997
616.1'32075--dc21
DNLM/DLC
for Library of Congress   97-29563
                                                                CIP

British Library Cataloguing in Publication Data
Semple, Peter
        An atlas of hypertension. – 2nd ed. – (The encyclopedia
of visual medicine series)
        I. Hypertension
        I. Title II. Lindop, George B.M., 1945–
        616.1'32
ISBN 1-85070-949-1

Published in the USA by
The Parthenon Publishing Group Inc.
One Blue Hill Plaza
PO Box 1564, Pearl River
New York 10965, USA

Published in the UK and Europe by
The Parthenon Publishing Group Limited
Casterton Hall, Carnforth
Lancs. LA6 2LA, UK

Copyright © 1998 Parthenon Publishing Group

Printed and bound in Spain by
T.G. Hostench, S.A.

Contents

Foreword

I have just finished reading *An Atlas of Hypertension* by Peter Semple and George Lindop.

The charm of this concise volume is its plain language and its simplicity as it surveys the complex hypertension landscape and defines the various different forms of hypertensive disease. The book also provides companion information on how to recognize and diagnose these hypertensive syndromes.

For those who are interested in pursuing causal mechanisms and clinical nuances in greater depth, a bibliography is provided.

This atlas should be a most valuable primary reference source for all clinicians interested in understanding high blood pressure, its natural history and its pathological consequences.

John H. Laragh
New York

Acknowledgements

The authors are grateful to the following colleagues who have kindly contributed some of their slides to this new edition:

Dr Grant Baxter, Department of Radiology, and
Dr David Davies, Department of Medicine and
  Therapeutics, The Western Infirmary,
  Glasgow; and
Dr Marie Callaghan, Department of Radiology,
  Law Hospital, Carluke, Lanarkshire.

Preface

In preparing this new edition of *An Atlas of Hypertension*, we were initially somewhat skeptical that there was enough that was new in the field of hypertension to justify the project. We were soon pleasantly surprised to discover that there have been so many new imaging systems and advances in clinical practice since the beginning of the decade.

Better quality and much less invasive methods of imaging the renal arteries, and advances in interventional radiology have transformed the investigation and treatment of atherosclerotic renovascular disease. Furthermore, the use of endovascular stents as an adjunct to percutaneous angioplasty has greatly increased the scope of the procedure, especially by allowing treatment of lesions at the ostia of the renal arteries.

The dissemination of accurate methods of non-invasive ambulatory monitoring of blood pressure has made it possible to recognize patients with arterial pressures that require treatment more quickly and with greater accuracy. When combined with sensitive methods of quantifying left ventricular hypertrophy such as echocardiography and magnetic resonance imaging, the selection of those requiring treatment can be even further refined.

Clinical trials have validated many aspects of the multiple-risk approach to treatment of patients with hypertension, and there is now an appreciation of the need to treat cholesterol and lipid levels and / or carbohydrate intolerance in many patients who have raised blood pressures, and a better understanding of those most likely to benefit from antihypertensive drugs. There is a growing body of evidence to support a more aggressive approach to blood pressure-lowering in patients with all forms of diabetes mellitus to prevent nephropathy, and micro- and macrovascular complications.

For clinicians involved in the detection and management of hypertension and other risk factors, the main challenge now is to implement what is already known and currently available. Doubts as to the efficacy of treating hypertension even in older patients have been largely dispelled. The text of this atlas has been almost completely rewritten, and it is our hope that busy clinicians engaged in the treatment of hypertension in both primary and secondary care will find this revised volume useful.

Peter F. Semple
George B.M. Lindop
Glasgow

Section 1   A Review of Hypertension

Introduction

Detection and control of hypertension are the key to preventing stroke, but the goal of attaining normal blood pressures without side-effects is still not consistently achieved.

Overwhelming evidence supports the concept that blood pressure in the population is a continuously distributed variable, bearing a graded relationship to risk of vascular events, so that any definition of hypertension is, by necessity, arbitrary. The line dividing 'normal' from 'high' blood pressures is often set at 140 / 90 mmHg, although definitions vary. By most criteria, approximately 10–20% of adults will develop raised levels of blood pressure by the time they are middle-aged.

High blood pressure is most closely associated with an increased risk of stroke which is almost completely reversed if satisfactory control of blood pressure is achieved with drugs. The correlation between blood pressure and risk of coronary events is not as close as for stroke, and the evidence that this risk is reduced by treatment is still less well established.

High blood pressure recordings at initial screening tend to fall somewhat if repeated over weeks or months. This is thought to be a reflection of both an attenuation of the alarm reaction and a statistical phenomenon known as regression to the mean. As a method of diagnosis, monitoring of office or clinic blood pressures over relatively long periods of time is increasingly tending to be replaced by either ambulatory measurements taken over 24 h or home monitoring of blood pressure using semi-automatic devices.

Inherited factors are important in the pathogenesis of the most common form of high blood pressure, namely, primary or essential hypertension. The specific genes associated with the condition have not yet been identified, but there are likely to be several. Other factors, such as obesity, insulin resistance, dietary sodium intake, stress and excessive alcohol intake, interact with the genetic substrate.

Only around 5% or less of all hypertensive patients have a recognizable cause of their hypertension. In such cases of so-called secondary hypertension, the hypertension is most often due to underlying renal or renovascular disease, but other, less common, causes include syndromes of corticosteroid excess such as primary aldosteronism, and pheochromocytoma and coarctation of the aorta.

Severe hypertension may develop into an accelerated or malignant form but, in developed countries, the incidence has declined steeply in recent years. The clinical diagnosis of malignant hypertension is relatively easy in the presence of bilateral flame-shaped retinal hemorrhages. Such fundal changes are accompanied by fibrinoid necrosis in the arterioles of the kidney which is typical of the condition. Moderately raised blood pressure does not usually give rise to symptoms unless a cardiovascular event such as stroke or myocardial infarction has occurred.

High blood pressure has long been recognized as a factor that accelerates the development of atherosclerosis and causes coronary artery disease. In such cases, blood pressure then interacts positively with other factors such as blood levels of cholesterol, cigarette-smoking and obesity.

Because treatment trials in hypertension have shown a somewhat disappointing impact on myocardial infarction compared with stroke and heart failure, there has been a tendency towards an integrated approach to correct risk factors in the individual patient. Various tables have also been devised that attempt to quantify individual risk and to facilitate identification of the patients most likely to benefit from drug treatment of high concentrations of blood cholesterol.

Target organs

Brain

The risk of stroke is directly related to arterial pressure, and this graded relationship appears to be maintained even within the normal range of diastolic blood pressure (DBP). Meta-analysis of nine prospective observational studies confirmed that there is no convincing evidence of a 'threshold' level of DBP at which risk begins. In general, with sustained increases in DBP of 5, 7.5 and 10 mmHg, there are corresponding increases in stroke risk of 34%, 46% and 56%, respectively. Of the factors that predict stroke, blood pressure is dominant, although other independent risk factors have been identified and include smoking, obesity and plasma levels of fibrinogen.

The incidence of stroke remains particularly low in some underdeveloped countries where the average DBP may be only 60 mmHg. In China, Japan and parts of Africa, high blood pressure and stroke are common, but coronary artery disease is relatively infrequent. This discrepancy, at least in the Far East, is probably due to differences in the prevailing levels of blood cholesterol and low-density lipoprotein (LDL).

Just over 10% of all clinical strokes are caused by cerebral hemorrhage. Hemorrhages in hypertension are caused by rupture of microaneurysms which develop on the short penetrating branches of the main cerebral arteries. Such small aneurysms have been identified on arteries 50–200 μm in diameter principally at sites of branching, and are particularly frequently seen in the distribution of the lateral striate artery. The density of lesions tends to be highest in the putamen, globus pallidus, caudate nucleus, thalamus, external capsule and basis pontis. Hemorrhage into the putamen is especially frequent, and presents as weakness of the contralateral face, arm and leg, and is almost invariably accompanied by hyperreflexia at an early stage. Large lesions cause hemisensory loss and hemianopia with conjugate deviation of the eyes, reduced consciousness and aphasia or visuospatial neglect.

Another brain lesion associated with uncontrolled hypertension is a small infarct which evolves into a slit-like space or lacune 0.5–15 mm in diameter. These small deep infarcts are often undetectable on computed tomography (CT), and are the result of occlusion of one of the same perforating arteries that rupture in hypertensive cerebral hemorrhage. The arteries immediately proximal to small infarcts show segmental disorganization of the vessel wall, possibly resulting from mechanical disruption of the intima and insudation of plasma constituents. Such changes are seen in small arteries that are close to high-pressure arteries, but not in vessels of the same caliber at more remote sites. The relative underdevelopment of the muscle and elastic tissue layers of these particular small brain arteries may contribute to their vulnerability. Intraluminal pressures may also be higher in these arteries than in those of similar diameter elsewhere because of their shorter lengths.

Lacunar infarcts resulting from small-vessel disease probably account for up to 20% of ischemic strokes in the developed countries and most usually present as episodes of pure motor hemiparesis, pure sensory stroke or ataxic hemiparesis. Symptoms may evolve progressively over a period of 24–48 h. Because subcortical white matter is involved, there are no signs of cortical dysfunction such as dysphasia, neglect, agnosia or apraxia. Transient ischemic attacks may also occur. It is not difficult to imagine that the incidences of hemorrhage and lacunar infarction are greatly reduced by effective treatment of chronic hypertension.

Most strokes in Western populations are due to atheromatous disease often affecting extracranial vessels, especially the origin of the internal carotid artery. This predilection to atheroma is probably explained by the turbulent blood flow at a point of arterial bifurcation causing alterations in endothelial function. Atheroma most often causes cerebral infarction in the distribution of the middle cerebral artery, and large infarcts may become hemorrhagic after reperfusion. Vascular occlusion is initiated by rupture of the fibrous cap of an atherosclerotic plaque with superimposed thrombosis. In some instances, artery-to-artery embolism is the predominant mechanism of transient ischemic attacks (TIAs) in carotid artery stenosis.

The velocity of blood flow in narrowed vessels is increased, and this acceleration may be detected by Doppler ultrasonography in combination with a two-dimensional image of the structures referred to as the duplex method. Color flow imaging is now routine and refinements such as power Doppler have emerged. Most TIAs in the territory of a stenosed internal carotid artery are caused by atheroembolism with resultant hemiparesis or amaurosis fugax. In these cases, the fragmented emboli can sometimes be visualized as refractile cholesterol-rich deposits at points of bifurcation of the retinal arterioles.

Clinical trials have clearly shown that drug treatment of hypertension reduces the incidence of fatal and non-fatal stroke by around 40%, and benefit appears to accrue after relatively short periods of blood pressure reduction. The results of outcome trials have not differentiated between hemorrhage, lacunar stroke and atherothrombotic infarction. Antihypertensive drug treatment in combination with antithrombotic measures has a place in the secondary prevention of stroke, but caution should be exercised in the period immediately after stroke because cerebral autoregulation tends to be impaired. Aspirin is now universally prescribed for secondary prevention of ischemic stroke unless there is a specific contraindication. Other antiplatelet agents, such as clopidogrel and dipyridamole, may also be effective, but all have the potential to worsen intracerebral hemorrhage. In the presence of a critical proximal arterial stenosis, antihypertensive drugs may provoke ischemic events especially in the boundary zones between arterial territories. Symptomatic carotid stenosis is best treated by endarterectomy.

Retina

Accelerated or malignant hypertension is defined as the finding of bilateral retinal hemorrhages, which tend to be flame-shaped or linear, together with a DBP that is usually > 120 mmHg. In the days before effective drug treatment of hypertension, around 80% of patients with malignant hypertension died within a year. Blurred vision is a common presenting complaint; other symptoms include morning headache which tends to be occipital, exertional dyspnea and weight loss. Bleeding, such as epistaxis or hemospermia, may occur. Earlier and more effective treatment of hypertension has rendered encephalopathy with obtundation and seizures very rare, although the condition is still seen in children and in parts of Africa where malignant hypertension remains a major problem.

Papilledema indicates edema of the brain due to raised intracranial pressure but, in itself, does not appear to identify patients with a prognosis that is significantly different from those who have retinal hemorrhages and 'cottonwool' spots. A diagnosis of malignant hypertension cannot be sustained if hemorrhages are unilateral because of the possibility of confusion with central or branch retinal-vein occlusion.

So-called cottonwool spots are areas of infarction of the nerve-fiber layer of the retina. In contrast, refractile 'hard exudates' are caused by the escape of plasma from permeable small vessels with deposition of lipid in the retina. Hard exudates tend to cluster at the macula and may give rise to an appearance described as a macular 'star', and are often seen in the resolving phase of hypertensive retinopathy. Hemorrhages, cottonwool spots and papilledema clear after only a few weeks of antihypertensive therapy, but hard exudates may persist for several months.

Hypertension causes narrowing of the retinal arterioles, which may show focal spasm in more severe cases. The normal ratio of artery:vein diameter is >3:4. Changes in the light reflex reflect hyalinization of the vessel wall or arteriosclerosis, and occur with hypertension and increasing age; grading is difficult in clinical practice. More severe grades of high blood pressure cause 'silver wiring' of the arterioles which appear to nip the retinal veins at crossing points that tend to become right-angled.

Heart

Left ventricular hypertrophy

An increase in peripheral vascular resistance is characteristic of the established phase of hypertension. Left ventricular work is increased as a consequence and results in concentric hypertrophy. Although changes in cardiac geometry tend to normalize wall stresses during systole, they reduce compliance, causing diastolic dysfunction, and increase myocardial oxygen demand.

A hypertrophic ventricle initially functions well but, in the later stages, there is progressive dilatation associated with a steep decline in performance. Myocyte ischemia may be caused by the combined effects of poor perfusion due to diastolic dysfunction and increased demand for oxygen from hypertrophied myocytes. There is usually an accompanying reduction in capillary density or rarefaction and an increase in the diffusion distance for oxygen. Coronary flow reserve, which is the difference between normal flow rate and flow rate at maximum dilatation, is reduced in the hypertrophied ventricle and flow to the subendocardial zone is particularly jeopardized.

Part of the reduction in compliance of the left ventricle in hypertension is caused by deposition of increased collagen which may not be reversed by antihypertensive treatment. The hypertrophied left ventricle becomes stiff and may not be adequately filled during diastole so that a serious decline in cardiac output may ensue if atrial fibrillation removes the active phase of ventricular filling. Echocardiography and magnetic resonance imaging (MRI) are considerably more sensitive than electrocardiography (ECG) in detecting ventricular hypertrophy in hypertension.

Severe left ventricular hypertrophy (LVH) predisposes to serious ventricular arrhythmias and sudden death. The Framingham Study has shown that LVH is an independent risk factor. During 12 years of follow-up, the mortality of patients with LVH, as determined by ECG criteria, was 16%, rising to 60% in the presence of a concurrent strain 'pattern'.

Coronary artery disease

In Europe and North America, high blood pressure is also a major risk factor for coronary artery disease and sudden cardiac death. As with stroke, the relationship between blood pressure and coronary events is probably continuous across the whole blood pressure distribution so that those in the highest quintile of the distribution have an incidence about five times greater than those in the lowest quintile. The event rate in the lowest part of the distribution is generally rather low and variable between studies, but some workers have proposed that low DBP in treated hypertension precipitates coronary events. This putative J-shaped relationship to risk continues to be a subject for debate.

High blood pressure accelerates atherosclerosis, which is also highly dependent on blood levels of cholesterol, LDL cholesterol and other lipoproteins, such as lipoprotein (a), as well as cigarette-smoking, obesity and diabetes mellitus. In Japan and China, where populations have low cholesterol levels, the incidence of coronary artery disease is relatively low, although the stroke mortality rate in China is currently around twice that in the United Kingdom.

Few individual trials of drug treatment of hypertension have shown significant reductions in myocardial infarction or coronary events. The reasons for this discrepancy with stroke have been much debated. Drug treatments appear to reduce slightly the incidence of congestive heart failure, probably as a reflection of the prevention or reversal of LVH.

Various explanations for the failure to reduce the rate of coronary events have been proposed. For example, it is possible that the time course of the effects of lowering blood pressure on atherosclerosis is different from the time course of small-vessel disease. Indeed, most treatment trials have been of relatively short duration (3–5 years) and have terminated at the point where a significant reduction in stroke is attained. Meta-analysis of the results of all the major trials of treatment in mild-to-moderate hypertension suggests a significant reduction in coronary event rate of about 14%. It is disappointing that there is still a paucity of outcome of clinical trials for angiotensin-converting enzyme (ACE) inhibitors or angiotensin-receptor antagonist and calcium antagonist drugs.

Aorta and arteries

In hypertension, the small arteries develop medial thickening and arteriosclerosis is accelerated. The change in small-vessel geometry results in an increase in wall-to-wall lumen ratio and enhances the pressor response to vasoconstrictor substances. This is often described as the 'vascular amplifier' and may have a role in aggravating hypertension. The possible causes of a change in wall-to-lumen ratio are smooth muscle cell hypertrophy, hyperplasia or rearrangement of the same cells around a reduced lumen, described as remodelling. In hypertension in humans, remodelling may predominate, but the relative importance of the three factors remains the subject of debate.

Circulating or local vasoactive agents such as angiotensin II also have growth-promoting effects on smooth muscle and, conversely, growth factors such as platelet-derived growth factor (PDGF) may be potent vasoconstrictors. This so-called humoral amplifier may act in concert with the vascular amplifier to promote structural change. In contrast, vasodilators such as nitric oxide usually inhibit cell growth, and may reduce pressure by both direct and indirect mechanisms. Arterial structure is affected by local and circulating factors, and it has become increasingly evident that the vascular endothelium responds to hemodynamic stimuli by producing vasoactive substances, some of which also modulate smooth muscle cell growth.

Medial hypertrophy evolves towards arteriosclerosis, including so-called 'hyaline' sclerosis of arterioles as well as sclerosis of larger arteries. Age-related changes resemble those seen in long-standing hypertension. Hyalin is restricted to arterioles and the smallest arteries, and is concentrated in vessels of the kidney, brain, retina, spleen and gut with relative sparing of heart, skeletal muscle and skin.

In the brain, heart and kidneys, blood flow remains constant despite wide variations in arterial pressure, a phenomenon known as autoregulation. In hypertension, loss of arterial compliance due to arteriosclerosis causes the autoregulation curve to be shifted to the right so that vasodilatation and 'flow reserve' are compromised. This shift probably partly explains the susceptibility of older patients to cerebral infarction when there is overtreatment of hypertension.

In the aorta and other large elastic arteries, hypertension and aging cause dilatation, lengthening and loss of compliance. Unfolding of the ascending aorta is often seen on plain chest radiography and severe dilatation of the aortic root sometimes causes aortic regurgitation. Loss of elasticity accounts for the relatively greater increase of systolic blood pressure (SBP) rather than DBP with age and causes pulse-wave velocity to increase. The effect of this increased velocity is that the reflected wave from the periphery reaches the heart in systole rather than diastole, thereby increasing cardiac workload and promoting ventricular hypertrophy. It is now clear that isolated systolic hypertension in the elderly benefits from treatment with antihyper-

tensive drugs, especially diuretic-based regimens. Severe hypertension causes an increase in glycosaminoglycan in the aortic media and predisposes to the relatively rare complication of aortic dissection.

Kidneys

Renal failure often develops in patients with malignant hypertension, but is relatively rare in non-malignant hypertension, perhaps because of more effective treatment. In the era before antihypertensive drugs, death from renal failure in malignant hypertension was commonplace. African-Americans have a high prevalence of renal impairment caused by hypertension compared with Caucasians.

Malignant hypertension causes fibrinoid necrosis of the small arteries and arterioles in the kidney, especially in the afferent glomerular arterioles, but also affecting small radial arteries. Fibrin in the vessel wall is the result of plasmatic vasculosis, a process which allows plasma proteins, including fibrinogen, to gain access to the media. This is accompanied by necrosis of smooth muscle cells and thrombosis of the lumen, leading to obliteration of the glomeruli, and the presence of red cells and red casts in the urine. Intimal proliferation, which is most prominent in the radial arteries, leads to the characteristic 'onion-skin' appearance, which may represent a healing response to endothelial cell injury. The glomeruli undergo focal necrosis, and glomerular capillaries may rupture into Bowman's space and the renal tubules to cause a 'flea-bitten' appearance to the surface of the kidney. Fibrin deposition in blood vessels occasionally causes fragmentation of circulating red blood cells, resulting in so-called microangiopathic hemolytic anemia with thrombocytopenia.

Lowering arterial pressure usually stabilizes renal function if renal impairment is due to hypertensive nephrosclerosis, and also reduces the rate of functional deterioration in many chronic renal conditions. Autosomal-dominant polycystic disease is an example where hypertension is an early feature. The cause of progressive renal failure in kidney disease is not well understood, although overperfusion of the reduced number of residual nephrons may be the main pathogenetic mechanism.

Diabetes mellitus

Diabetic nephropathy is a major cause of end-stage renal disease in the developed countries with an average survival after the onset of persistent proteinuria of only 5–10 years. Treatment of hypertension slows the rate of loss of renal function and ACE inhibitors appear to be more effective in this context than beta-blockers or the dihydropyridine calcium antagonists, perhaps because of specific effects on glomerular hemodynamics. In type I (insulin-dependent) diabetes, hypertension tends to develop in parallel with nephropathy, and a factor that promotes proteinuria and deterioration of renal function. Treatment with ACE inhibitors clearly reduces proteinuria and non-dihydropyridine calcium antagonists, such as verapamil, have similar effects. It is not yet clear whether angiotensin-receptor antagonists share this property.

Other aspects of treatment, such as more intensive control of blood sugar, also reduce the risk of developing micro- or macroalbuminuria. This was best demonstrated in the Diabetes Control and Complications Trial. The use of ACE inhibitors in diabetics may be extended to lower levels of blood pressure than in primary hypertension. In patients with more advanced renal impairment due to diabetic nephropathy, there is an increased risk of atherosclerosis and renovascular disease so that ACE inhibitors have the potential to impair function.

In type II (non-insulin-dependent) diabetes, the relationship with hypertension may be somewhat different. It is clear from many epidemiological surveys that there is an association between hypertension, obesity, insulin resistance and type II diabetes that is independent of nephropathy, and there may be a common genetic predisposition. Up to 25% of patients with type II diabetes develop microalbuminuria, and hypertension worsens proteinuria and accelerates renal impairment. As in type I diabetes, microalbuminuria may be an indication for treatment with an ACE inhibitor and the thresholds for blood pressure treatment may be lower than in primary hypertension. The presence of type II diabetes is a factor in the choice of antihypertensive drug. Thiazide diuretics are not drugs of first choice, and ACE inhibitors and non-dihydropyridine calcium antagonists tend to be preferable to beta-blockers. Alpha-blockers also do not impair carbohydrate or lipid metabolism.

Measurement of blood pressure

For routine clinical purposes, the mercury sphygmomanometer remains a robust, reliable and accurate instrument for measurement of arterial pressure. Aneroid devices tend to be less reliable and should be checked at least once a year against a mercury instrument. Such a check is conveniently made using a 'Y' connection between the tubing of the two instruments. There is now a wide variety of electronic machines available for home blood pressure monitoring, although the standards of accuracy vary considerably.

Accuracy

There are important points to observe if accurate measurements are to be obtained by indirect methods. The first is the vexed question of cuff size, which has exercised minds since Riva-Rocci described the first instrument in 1896. Cuffs that are too small overestimate pressure and the converse is also true. There is general agreement that the bladder should almost encircle the arm and have a width that is 40% of the circumference of the arm. Current recommendations in the UK are to use a 35×12.5-cm cuff for adults with 35–42-cm arm circumferences. With arm circumferences <35 cm, a smaller bladder (18×8 cm) should be used and, for obese arms, a larger cuff is required.

It has become apparent that training in the correct use of the mercury sphygmomanometer is essential to reduce error. In previous years, instruction was often minimal. Methods of reducing observer error include formal instruction combined with the use of videos, films or audio cassette tapes.

Mercury sphygmomanometers should be checked every 6 months in hospital use and every year otherwise. Problems are relatively infrequent, but include loss of mercury so that the meniscus is not at zero when the cuff is deflated and black deposits of oxidized mercury on the inner surface of the glass that obscure the meniscus. Occasionally, there is a leak in the system so that the rate of descent of the column of mercury is >2 mm / s. It should always be possible to inflate the bladder to a pressure >200 mmHg in less than 5 s. The Velcro® on a cuff may wear out so that there is poor apposition of bladder to arm.

Measurements of pressure should be made with the arm supported at heart level. At the initial clinical assessment of a patient, blood pressures should be measured in both arms sequentially. If the difference between the arms is >20 / 10 mmHg, then simultaneous measurements of both arms using two instruments should be taken and the arm that gives higher values should be used for subsequent monitoring. In patients in the last trimester of pregnancy in the recumbent position, there is an increase in pulse rate and narrowing of the pulse pressure due to sympathetic activation caused by reduced venous return. Placing the patient in the lateral position minimizes the reflex activation.

Blood pressures are normally recorded to the nearest 2 mmHg. In most circumstances, the DBP is measured at Korotkoff phase V, the point at which sounds disappear. In cases where there is a wide pulse pressure due to aortic regurgitation or rapid run-off into the peripheral circulation, phase V may continue to 0 mmHg. In such an event, the DBP should be recorded at phase IV, where there is muffling of the heart sounds.

Ambulatory monitoring

Non-invasive ambulatory monitoring of blood pressure is available in most centers for diagnosis and assessing the adequacy of control of hypertension with antihypertensive treatment. The technique provides a profile of blood pressures over 24 or 48 h with information on diurnal patterns and nocturnal levels of blood pressure. Although there are not yet sufficient epidemiological data to relate levels to morbidity and mortality, studies are underway to address some of these questions. At present, normal values tend to be defined on the basis of cross-sectional studies and meta-analyses. It has been proposed that normal daytime values may be as low as 126 / 83 or as high as 150 / 95 mmHg, but there is no current consensus of opinion.

The technique has value in detecting 'white-coat' hypertension and identifying those who do not show a nocturnal dip. The white-coat effect may be a factor in 20% or more of patients with hypertension diagnosed by office or clinic blood pressure recording. It has been further proposed that the term 'white-coat hypertension' should be reserved for patients who have persistently high clinic blood pressure readings, but normal ambulatory values whereas the term 'white-coat phenomenon' can be reserved for those who have a tendency for higher values during the first 1–2 h of ambulatory recording. It has also not yet been ascertained that white-coat hypertension has an entirely benign prognosis. What is well established is that the correlation between ambulatory blood pressure and LVH is closer with ambulatory than with office recordings and, thus, the technique is useful in patients who have borderline hypertension.

On occasions, ambulatory monitoring has been useful in detecting fluctuating hypertension in pheochromocytoma, and a lack of diurnal variation sometimes points to a secondary cause. In patients with high clinic recordings despite treatment, ambulatory recordings may demonstrate whether blood pressure control is truly poor. Blood pressure-profile changes over 24 h also provide insights into antihypertensive drug effects and facilitate calculation of trough-to-peak ratios for individual agents.

The issue of accuracy is pertinent and, thus, it is essential that the instruments available on the market should meet validation criteria such as the British Hypertension Society protocol. General experience with several systems suggests that accuracy is not maintained at high levels of blood pressure, although the practical significance of this type of error is likely to be minimal. At present, a weakness of all systems is the intermittent nature of the measurement. More detailed and accurate profiles can be obtained by intra-arterial methods, but their invasive nature excludes them from routine practice. It is already clear that ambulatory measurements are superior to clinic values in terms of prognosis, but a definitive statement of their value must await the completion of longitudinal studies.

Investigation of secondary hypertension

Renovascular disease

Renovascular disease is generally uncommon if sought in asymptomatic patients with mild-to-moderate hypertension in young adults and the middle-aged. The prevalence in cross-sectional surveys in the developed countries is usually around 3% or less. Certain groups are at high risk of atheromatous renal artery stenosis, notably patients with peripheral vascular disease wherein approximately 30% of patients have unilateral, and around 10% have bilateral, renal artery stenosis. Bilateral disease may comprise stenosis on one side and an occlusion contralaterally. With stenosis >75% of luminal diameter, there is a risk of arterial occlusion ranging from 8% to 16% over 2 to 3 years.

Deterioration of renal function after treatment with an ACE inhibitor or angiotensin-receptor antagonist is now a relatively common cause of presentation. Renovascular disease may also be suspected where there is an unexplained deterioration in control of blood pressure with drug treatment, especially if such treatment does not include an ACE inhibitor or angiotensin-receptor antagonist. If there is an abdominal aortic aneurysm or internal carotid artery stenosis, there may be concurrent renal artery atherosclerosis. Although not often encountered nowadays, patients with malignant or accelerated hypertension are also more likely to have renovascular disease, especially if the condition develops in a patient >50 years old.

For patients <40 years of age, renovascular disease is uncommon except with fibromuscular dysplasia. This rare condition should be suspected if a woman, especially a cigarette-smoker, develops severe hypertension with no family history of high blood pressure or stroke. Plasma renin activity is usually high in the untreated state and normalization of blood pressure after treatment with an ACE inhibitor or angiotensin-receptor antagonist is characteristic. The typical appearances are relatively easy to identify on angiography, and there may be a 'beaded' segment of artery where areas of arterial narrowing are interspersed with areas of dilatation. Other arteries of similar caliber, such as the carotid or mesenteric artery, may also be affected. The condition predisposes to arterial dissection which, in the case of the renal artery, may present with flank pain and hematuria.

Fibromuscular disease responds particularly well to revascularization by angioplasty or surgery, providing that technical success has been achieved. Blood pressures are normalized in >50% of cases. This contrasts with the response rate in atheromatous renal artery disease where cure occurs in <20% of patients treated. As with most forms of hypertension, the factors which tend to predict a poor blood pressure response to revascularization include overall impairment of renal function, reduced kidney size and long-term hypertension.

The low prevalence of renovascular disease in the general hypertensive population at around 3% indicates that screening tests must have a high degree of both sensitivity and specificity. The best functional tests available miss around 30% of cases and give a positive yield on arteriography of approximately 1 in 5 cases. Of the functional tests available, rapid-sequence intravenous urography is now obsolete. Measurement of plasma renin activity 1 h after administration of captopril has a sensitivity of 84% and a specificity of 93%, but may be compromised in many patients by antihypertensive drug treatment.

Renal scintigraphy after captopril is one of the best non-invasive screening methods, but diethylenetriamine pentaacetic acid (DTPA) scintigraphy has a sensitivity of only 70–80% with a 90% specificity, and the widely used mercaptoacetyl triglycine (MAG-3) technique is probably less sensitive. Doppler ultrasonography of the main renal arteries with contrast is sometimes useful, but is highly operator-dependent. Around 8% of arteries may not be visualized and approximately 20% of kidneys are supplied by more than one artery. Pulsatility of an interlobar artery distal to stenosis can be measured by Doppler technology, but is inadequate for screening, although it may be useful in detecting restenosis after angioplasty. Magnetic resonance angiography and spiral computed tomography (CT) both show promise, but only relatively small series of patients have been reported at present.

Some centers, including that of the authors, only screen those patients in whom there is a high index of clinical suspicion. Intra-arterial digital subtraction angiography using a 4-F catheter and an aortic flush injection of contrast is the best means of visualizing a renal artery stenosis. Intravenous injection methods require larger doses of contrast and adequate definition of the renal arteries may not be attained, especially in cases of reduced cardiac output. Renal vein renin sampling after captopril stimulation is sometimes useful in diagnosis and may have value in predicting a successful outcome after revascularization. Suppression of renin secretion from the kidney contralateral to a stenosis may also be of significance.

Conservation or improvement of renal function is often a reason for investigation and treatment, especially now that ostial stenoses due to aortic plaque can be treated with vascular endoprostheses. There have also been occasional anecdotal reports of beneficial effects of treating renal artery stenosis in patients with heart failure. Successful revascularization or placement of a stent may prevent kidney loss due to thrombosis superimposed on severe stenosis, but controlled trials have not yet been carried out.

If angioplasty achieves revascularization of a kidney, it may be possible to use an ACE inhibitor or angiotensin-receptor antagonist with a reduced risk of worsening renal failure, but careful monitoring of renal function remains mandatory. The complication rate of angioplasty and stent placement in experienced hands is low, although 5–10% of cases may develop groin hematoma. Arteriography or angioplasty in patients with severe atherosclerosis may precipitate cholesterol embolism, which can cause deterioration in renal function, abdominal pain, livedo reticularis or ischemic lesions of the toes.

Surgery for renal artery stenosis has been largely superseded by percutaneous balloon angioplasty. Endovascular stents allow treatment of ostial lesions and cases where elastic recoil is a problem. Restenosis may be a problem in up to 15% of treated patients at 2 years, but the incidence after stent replacement may not be as high. Despite the technical advances in investigation and treatment of renovascular disease, only a few controlled clinical trials have compared revascularization with medical treatment.

Renal hypertension

Most renal diseases that impair kidney function cause high blood pressure. Patients with hypertension while undergoing renal replacement treatment often have LVH.

The type of glomerulonephritis that is most often encountered in blood pressure clinics is IgA nephropathy or Berger's disease. The condition is so-called because immunocytochemistry of renal tissue shows that mesangial deposition of IgA is a prominent feature. The disease appears to be ubiquitous, but is perhaps less common in Northern Europe and the USA than in Southern Europe and Asia. Some patients present with frank hematuria, but hypertension associated with persistent microscopic hematuria and mild proteinuria may bring the condition to the attention of physicians treating hypertension. The condition tends to affect men and progression to end-stage renal failure may be relatively slow.

Most patients with chronic renal failure have high blood pressure caused largely by a combination of volume expansion due to retention of sodium and water, and activation of the renin–angiotensin system. Control of blood pressure often necessitates multiple drug regimens, including loop diuretics such as frusemide, which may need to be given in large doses. Restriction of dietary sodium intake to around 50 mmol / day or less may be a helpful measure.

In patients undergoing dialysis treatment, blood pressure control is more readily achieved with the continuous ambulatory peritoneal technique than with intermittent peritoneal dialysis or hemo-

dialysis. Erythropoietin treatment of anemia tends to increase arterial pressure in parallel with the rise in hematocrit and blood viscosity.

Chronic renal disease is the most common cause of high blood pressure in children and young adults. Reflux nephropathy is a particularly important cause of high blood pressure in females in this age group and may present as severe or malignant hypertension. Disease is often bilateral, but unilateral reflux with renal scarring and unilateral renin secretion is sometimes seen. Hypertension may then be cured or greatly improved by nephrectomy, provided that there is adequate function in the remaining kidney. Mild high blood pressure in children or young adults may be due to primary hypertension, but investigation to exclude renal disease is often appropriate in this age group. The rate of rise in blood pressure in adolescents is particularly marked if they are overweight.

Mineralocorticoid hypertension

Primary aldosteronism

Primary aldosteronism or Conn's syndrome is a much less common cause of high blood pressure than is renovascular hypertension. It most often affects women, and may present with symptoms of weakness and polyuria. The condition is usually first suspected after routine measurement of plasma electrolytes reveals concentrations indicative of hypokalemia, accompanied by a slight increase in the serum concentration of sodium. As hypokalemia may be intermittent, measurement of serum concentrations of potassium is not a good screening test, and serum potassium concentrations may be normal if dietary sodium intake is low.

Paralysis of skeletal muscle caused by severe hypokalemia is rare, but has been seen in patients who have primary aldosteronism after treatment with a thiazide or loop diuretic, and in subjects habituated to licorice.

In primary aldosteronism, there is a marked suppression of plasma renin activity or concentration except in patients treated with a diuretic or following a low-sodium diet. As a screening test, renin levels tend to be non-specific because nearly 30% of white hypertensives and a higher proportion of blacks have somewhat low renin values. The confounding effect of a diet of low-sodium content may be excluded by measuring urinary sodium excretion over 24 h and relating this value to the concurrent level of renin activity. Plasma renin activity also remains suppressed after ACE inhibitor treatment.

A diagnosis of primary aldosteronism is confirmed by high plasma concentrations of aldosterone in samples taken in the morning or increased urinary aldosterone excretion with marked suppression of plasma renin activity or concentration. An anomalous postural fall in plasma levels of aldosterone is sometimes present. In the presence of low levels of renin and angiotensin II, aldosterone secretion follows the diurnal rhythm of adrenocorticotropic hormone (ACTH) such that a component of the decrease observed after ambulation between 0800 and 1200 h may be due to the diurnal variation in ACTH. In cases of difficulty, measurement of the 18-hydroxylated steroids 18-hydroxycorticosterone and 18-hydroxycortisol may be helpful. Raised levels of 18-hydroxycortisol suggest autonomous secretion of aldosterone. Levels of these 18-hydroxylated steroids are less likely to be attenuated by hypokalemia compared with aldosterone.

Low plasma renin activity accompanied by low concentrations of aldosterone point to hypertension caused by another mineralocorticoid, either self-administered or endogenous. Some of the rare syndromes due to inherited deficiencies of the enzyme for corticosteroid biosynthesis cause mineralocorticoid hypertension with high levels of ACTH stimulating adrenal secretion of deoxy-corticosterone.

Once a biochemical diagnosis of primary aldosteronism is established, localization of an adenoma is the next step. Tumors are often visualized on CT or MRI, but small adenomas <1.5 cm in diameter may not be recognized. CT does not distinguish non-functioning adenomas from aldosteronomas. If a tumor >3 cm in diameter is identified, then malignancy should be suspected. Malignant renal tumors seldom present with mineralocorticoid hypertension and rarely, if ever, synthesize aldosterone, but some secrete other mineralocorticoids, notably deoxycorticosterone.

If an adenoma is suspected, then adrenal vein catheterization with measurement of aldosterone in adrenal venous blood is the most accurate way of confirming or establishing the diagnosis before surgery. However, this may be difficult on the right side. Seleno- or iodocholesterol scintigraphy, after a period of dexamethasone pretreatment, tends to give a high proportion of false negatives. A small proportion of patients (10–20%) have idiopathic aldosteronism without adenoma, although a tumor cannot be excluded unless adrenal venous sampling has been carried out. Differentiation of idiopathic aldosteronism from low-renin primary hypertension can also be difficult.

The initial treatment of primary aldosteronism is with potassium-sparing diuretics such as amiloride (10–40 mg / day), which corrects extracellular fluid volume expansion, reduces blood pressure and normalizes serum potassium. Spironolactone is an alternative to amiloride and may be used in doses of up to 300 mg / day. With spironolactone, there is a significant incidence of side-effects and there are concerns over the potential of large doses to cause breast cancer. For this reason, it is preferable not to use spironolactone in high doses for long-term treatment. The response of blood pressure to drug treatment tends to predict the effect of surgery.

Total exchangeable sodium, as measured by isotopic dilution, ranges from 105% to 120% of normal in untreated adenoma patients and falls to 100% or less after drug treatment or surgery. Plasma renin activity is a convenient index of extracellular fluid-volume status during drug treatment and of the dose of amiloride or spironolactone. The dose that controls blood pressure tends to reduce exchangeable sodium to below normal, which may reflect the relatively high prevalence of residual hypertension after surgery.

Blood pressure after surgery is normalized in only around 50% of patients. If renal function is impaired, then a satisfactory blood pressure response to medical treatment or surgery is much less likely. Extracellular volume expansion due to mineralocorticoids normally causes an increase in glomerular filtration rate so that creatinine clearance tends to fall after medical or surgical treatment unless renal function is impaired.

Other forms of mineralocorticoid hypertension

Syndromes caused by deficiency of the enzymes involved in cortisol biosynthesis, such as 17α-hydroxylase and 11β-hydroxylase, cause mineralocorticoid hypertension. 17α-Hydroxylase deficiency is accompanied by failure of sexual development as the enzyme is necessary for synthesis of sex steroids. 11β-Hydroxylase deficiency is accompanied by virilization in females or precocious puberty in males. In both syndromes, decreased cortisol secretion releases ACTH from feedback inhibition, resulting in excessive secretion of the mineralocorticoid deoxycorticosterone. A further extremely rare enzyme deficiency is 11β-hydroxysteroid deficiency, wherein cortisol to cortisone metabolism within the kidney and other tissues is reduced, thereby exposing the mineralocorticoid receptor to cortisol in high concentrations. This 'shuttle' enzyme normally protects the mineralocorticoid receptor from circulating cortisol and is inhibited by licorice and the licorice derivative carbenoxolone sodium.

Cushing's syndrome

Hypertension also occurs frequently in Cushing's syndrome, although the mechanism is not as clearly defined as in primary aldosteronism. Hypertension appears to occur most often in ACTH-mediated disease. Several factors may be involved in the pathogenesis, including activation of type I (mineralocorticoid) and type II (glucocorticoid) receptors by cortisol, and production of other hypertensinogenic steroids from the adrenal cortex. Hypokalemia is more likely if ACTH levels are particularly high, as in the ectopic syndrome. Cushing's syndrome due to an adrenal adenoma or carcinoma is relatively uncommon and accounts for around 10% of cases.

Hypertension in pituitary-dependent Cushing's disease usually responds to transsphenoidal hypophysectomy. Otherwise, hypertensive inpatients with Cushing's syndrome should be treated with conventional antihypertensive drugs, perhaps avoiding thiazide diuretics because of the risk of worsening glucose intolerance.

Pheochromocytoma

Pheochromocytoma is a rare cause of secondary hypertension which often causes problems in diagnosis. Routine screening in mild-to-moderate hypertension is not merited. Symptoms include paroxysmal headache, sweating and pallor. In some cases, hypertension may worsen with drug treatment especially if non-selective beta-blockers have been given.

Pheochromocytoma is often called the 'disease of 10%': around 10% are malignant, 10% are bilateral and 10% are extra-adrenal. Bilateral disease is almost invariable in type IIA multiple endocrine neoplasia, a Mendelian-dominant condition caused by a mutation in the RET proto-oncogene and associated with medullary carcinoma of the thyroid. The less common variant is type IIB where there are associated mucosal neuromas and skeletal deformities. Genetic screening with DNA probes can now identify carriers with a high degree of confidence. The Mendelian-dominant von Hippel–Lindau disease also predisposes to pheochromocytoma and renal carcinoma.

Diagnosis is best made from measurements of plasma and urine concentrations of norepinephrine (noradrenaline) and epinephrine (adrenaline). Plasma levels of catecholamines are almost invariably raised if hypertension is present when samples are taken. Suppression tests with clonidine provide the most sensitive method of diagnosis and easily distinguish raised plasma levels of catecholamines due to sympathoadrenal activation from raised levels caused by autonomous tumor secretion. Plasma levels of chromogranin A or neuropeptide Y, present in catecholamine storage vesicles, may be raised in pheochromocytoma, but have not found a role in routine diagnosis.

Tumors are usually located on CT; ultrasonography may not be sensitive enough to detect small lesions. In difficult cases, catheterization and selective sampling from the inferior vena cava and left renal vein for catecholamines may be helpful. Approximately 80% of tumors take up radioiodine (^{131}I)-labelled metaiodobenzylguanidine (MIBG), which may be helpful in scintigraphic localization of primary tumors and detection of metastatic deposits. Malignant tumors often metastasize to bone and isotope bone scans with an agent such as technetium 99m (^{99}Tc)-labelled methylene diphosphonate should be routine before consider-ing surgery. Some malignant tumors have been treated with therapeutic doses of ^{131}I-MIBG and a few, less differentiated, tumors have shown a useful response to cytotoxic drug treatment.

The long-acting non-competitive alpha-blocker phenoxybenzamine remains the drug of choice for controlling arterial pressure before surgery. Competitive blockers such as prazosin and labetalol have been somewhat disappointing in clinical practice. β_1-Adrenergic blockers may be used to control tachycardia. Most centers now use sodium nitroprusside for intraoperative control of blood pressure rather than the competitive blocker phentolamine, which has somewhat transient effects on blood pressure. Cardiac arrhythmias are generally prevented by careful control of pressure.

Hyperparathyroidism

There is an increased prevalence of hypertension in patients with primary hyperparathyroidism. Between 30% and 50% of affected patients have mild or moderately raised arterial pressure and some have LVH. The mechanism of the hypertension is not well understood, but may be related to the combined effects of extracellular hypercalcemia and excess parathyroid hormone.

The high blood pressure is not always corrected by parathyroid surgery, which may reflect an overlap with primary hypertension. In primary hypertension, a significant proportion of patients shows mild hypercalciuria and slightly raised levels of parathyroid hormone compared with controls who have normal blood pressure. This probably explains the increased incidence of renal calculus disease in patients with primary hypertension.

Acromegaly

Acromegaly is also associated with hypertension and there is evidence that, in these cases, the hypertension is related to increased body sodium content. Hypertrophic changes in cardiac and vascular muscle may also contribute to the raised blood pressure, which does not always respond to normalization of plasma levels of growth hormone.

Gestational hypertension

High blood pressure during pregnancy presents different problems. In normal pregnancy, blood pressure falls during the first trimester. Pre-eclamptic toxemia syndrome is diagnosed when hypertension with edema and proteinuria develops in late pregnancy associated with retardation of fetal growth. Thrombocytopenia and raised plasma concentrations of urate are characteristic, and intravascular volume is often reduced. In pre-eclampsia, blood pressures return rapidly to normal levels after delivery, but may occasionally persist a little longer.

In pregnancy-associated primary hypertension, high blood pressures are seen much earlier and respond to antihypertensive drug treatment. Methyldopa is still the preferred agent.

Estrogens, oral contraceptives and hormone replacement therapy

The commonly used estrogen-containing oral contraceptives (which contain 30 μg of estrogen) have mild pressor effects in many women. Therefore, monitoring of blood pressure before and after a prescription is routine. A few subjects show a marked pressor response and are probably the patients who eventually go on to develop raised blood pressure in later life. The obsolete 50 μg preparations produced pressor effects that were more marked. Progestogen-only pills do not appear to raise blood pressure and may be prescribed in women with hypertension. Low-dose estrogen treatment given to women after the decline of ovarian estrogen secretion in menopause does not raise blood pressure.

Coarctation of the aorta

Coarctation accounts for around 5–10% of all congenital cardiovascular anomalies and is a rare cause of hypertension. Aortic dissection, cerebral hemorrhage and heart failure are its associated complications. The condition is relatively common in women who have XO gonadal dysgenesis or Turner's syndrome.

In aortic coarctation, high blood pressure is most marked in the vessels of the upper body proximal to the lesion, the site of which is most often at or just beyond the insertion of the ligamentum arteriosum. A midsystolic murmur may be audible over the upper anterior chest and back, and aortic systolic murmurs frequently arise from a concurrent bicuspid aortic valve. Enlarged intercostal collateral vessels may be palpable around the chest and there may be overlying vascular bruits.

Pressure levels are much lower in the legs and may be determined with a thigh cuff. Coarctation is usually suspected when the femoral and other leg pulses are either absent, much reduced or delayed compared with pulses in the arm. MRI and spiral CT have proved to be useful techniques for diagnosis, supplemented by conventional angiography.

Aortic coarctation is usually detected in the first year of life. Delayed surgical correction of the coarctation leads to residual hypertension in 30–50% of patients who may require lifelong drug treatment. However, restenosis may also occur.

Interactions with lipids

Patients with raised blood pressure often have other risk factors for atherosclerotic arterial disease. Epidemiological studies have shown a tendency for these factors to cluster so that high blood pressure is associated with high plasma levels of cholesterol, obesity and abnormal glucose tolerance. Interventional trials with antihypertensive drugs alone have shown that the risk of coronary events is reduced, at best, by only one-third to one-half of expected.

Cigarette-smoking remains the major and most easily altered risk factor for coronary artery disease. It has been estimated that around 30% of all coronary deaths are probably caused by smoking. Population surveys have tended to show that smoking is either unrelated or inversely related to blood pressures. In trials of mild hypertension carried out by the Medical Research Council in the UK, the coronary event rate in male smokers was around twice the rate in non-smokers regardless of treatment, and the difference was emphasized in women. In general, outcome trials have shown that the difference between event rates in smokers with mild hypertension compared with non-smokers is greater than the difference in event rates between active antihypertensive treatment and placebo. Despite the absence of any correlation between smoking and blood pressure in population studies, there appears to be an association between cigarette-smoking and malignant hypertension which may be due to the increased prevalence of atherosclerotic renal artery stenosis.

Many prospective studies, including the Framingham study, carried out in the developed countries have shown that the risk of cardiovascular disease for a middle-aged man over a period of approximately 10 years shows a ten-fold gradient between those in the lowest quintile of distribution of plasma cholesterol and those in the highest quintile.

Across populations, the major difference in mortality rate due to ischemic heart disease in the Far East compared with Europe and North America appears to be related to differences in average cholesterol levels, as hypertension and cigarette-smoking are relatively common in both populations. In the Far East, there is an inverse and unexplained relationship between plasma levels of cholesterol and risk of cerebral hemorrhage. Compared with total cholesterol levels, the LDL subfraction is a better predictor of the presence of disease, and prediction is further refined if the ratio of LDL to high-density lipoprotein (HDL) cholesterol is used. The role of high triglyceride levels as an independent risk factor is still under debate, but is becoming more widely accepted.

The measurement and treatment of raised levels of total and LDL cholesterol with diet and drugs is central to the multiple risk factor approach that is increasingly being used to treat patients who have high blood pressure. Much effort has gone into defining the population subgroups who are at high coronary risk and who merit concurrent treatment with 3-hydroxy-3-methylglutaryl-CoA (HMG-CoA) reductase inhibitors (statins). Effects on lipids may be a consideration in the selection of antihypertensive drug treatment for the hyperlipidemic patient, although there are no outcome trials to validate such an approach.

Bibliography

Introduction

Alderman MH. Blood pressure management: Individualized treatment based on absolute risk and the potential for benefit. *Ann Intern Med* 1993; 119:329–35

Collins R, Peto R, MacMahon S, *et al.* Blood pressure and coronary heart disease. II. *Lancet* 1990;335:827–38

MacMahon S. Guidelines for antihypertensive therapy. *J Hypertens* 1996;14:691–3

MacMahon S, Peto R, Cutler J, *et al.* Blood pressure, stroke and coronary heart disease. I. *Lancet* 1990;335:765–74

Peart S, Brennan PJ, Broughton P, *et al.* Medical Research Council trial of treatment in older adults: Principal results. *Br Med J* 1992;304:505–12

Simpson FO. Guidelines for antihypertensive therapy: Problems with a strategy based on absolute cardiovascular risk. *J Hypertens* 1996;14: 683–9

Swales JD. Hypertension octet. Pharmacological treatment of hypertension. *Lancet* 1994;344:380–5

Systolic Hypertension in the Elderly Program (SHEP). Prevention of stroke by antihypertensive drug treatments: Final results from the Systolic Hypertension in the Elderly Program SHEP. *JAMA* 1991;265:3255–64

WHO–ISH Guidelines Subcommittee. 1993 Guidelines for the management of mild hypertension: Memorandum from a WHO–ISH meeting. *J Hypertens* 1993;11:905–18

Wolf PA, d'Agostino RB, Belanger AJ, Kannel WB. Probability of stroke: A risk profile from the Framingham Study. *Stroke* 1991;22:312–8

Target organs

Brain

Bamford J, Sandercock P, Dennis M, *et al.* Classification and natural history of clinically identifiable subtypes of cerebral infarction. *Lancet* 1991;337: 1521–6

Bogousslavsky J, Caplan L, eds. *Stroke Syndromes.* Cambridge: Cambridge University Press, 1995

Fisher CM. Lacunar infarcts: A review. *Cerebrovasc Dis* 1991;1:11–20

Kase CS, Caplan LR, eds. *Intracerebral Hemorrhage*. Boston: Butterworth–Heinemann, 1994

Skinhoj E, Strandgaard S. Pathogenesis of hypertensive encephalopathy. *Lancet* 1973;i:461–2

Retina

McGregor E, Isles CG, Lever AF, Murray GD. Retinal changes in malignant hypertension. *Br Med J* 1986;292:233–4

Heart

Left ventricular hypertrophy

Missouris CG, Forbat SM, Singer DRJ, *et al.* Echocardiography overestimates left ventricular mass: A comparative study with magnetic resonance imaging in patients with hypertension. *J Hypertens* 1996;4:1005–10

Hammond IW, Devereux RB, Alderman MH, *et al.* The prevalence and correlates of echocardiographic left ventricular hypertrophy among employed patients with uncomplicated hypertension. *J Am Coll Cardiol* 1986;7:639–50

McLenachan JM, Henderson E, Morris KL, Dargie HJ. Ventricular arrhythmias in patients with hypertensive LVH. *N Engl J Med* 1987;317:787–92

Nichols AB, Sciacca RR, Weiss MB, *et al.* Effect of left ventricular hypertrophy on myocardial blood flow and ventricular performance in systemic hypertension. *Circulation* 1980;62:329–40

Coronary artery disease

Anderson KM, Wilson PWF, Odell PW, Kannel WB. An updated coronary risk profile. A statement for health professionals. *Circulation* 1991;83:356–62

Collins R, Peto R, MacMahon S, *et al.* Blood pressure and coronary heart disease. II. *Lancet* 1990;335:827–38

Lichtenstein MJ, Shipley MJ, Rose G. Systolic and diastolic blood pressures as predictors of coronary heart disease mortality in the Whitehall study. *Br Med J* 1985;291:243–5

MacMahon S, Peto R, Cutler J, *et al.* Blood pressure, stroke and coronary heart disease. I. *Lancet* 1990;335:765–74

Aorta and arteries

Mulvany MJ. Resistance vessel structure in hypertension, growth or remodeling. *J Cardiovasc Pharmacol* 1993; 22(suppl 5):S44–7

O'Rourke MF, Kelly RP. Wave reflection in the systemic circulation, and its implication in ventricular function in man. *J Hypertens* 1993;11: 327–37

Kidneys

van Hooft IMS, Grobbee DE, Derckx FHM, *et al.* Renal hemodynamics and the renin–angiotensin–aldosterone system in normotensive subjects with hypertensive and normotensive parents. *N Engl J Med* 1991;324:1305–11

Janssen WMT, de Jong PE, de Zeeuw D. Hypertension and renal disease: Role of microalbuminuria. *J Hypertens* 1996;14(suppl 5):S173–7

Measurement of blood pressure

Petrie JC, O'Brien ET, Littler WA, de Swiet M, for the British Hypertension Society. Recommendations on blood pressure measurement. *Br Med J* 1986;293: 611–5

Ambulatory monitoring

Parati G, Omboni S, Mancia G. Difference between office and ambulatory blood pressure and response to antihypertensive treatment. *J Hypertens* 1996;14:791–7

Pickering TG. Which measures of blood pressure give the best prediction of target organ damage and prognosis? In Pickering TG, ed. *Ambulatory Monitoring and Blood Pressure Variability*. London: Science Press, 1991:13.1–15

Pickering TG, James GD, Boddie C, *et al*. How common is white-coat hypertension? *JAMA* 1988;259:225–8

Investigation of secondary hypertension

Renovascular hypertension

Blaufox MD, Middleton MM, Fine EG. In Laragh JH, Brenner BM, eds. *Hypertension: Pathophysiology, Diagnosis and Management*, 2nd edn. New York: Raven Press, 1996:2005–36

Bonelli FS, McKusick MA, Textor SC, *et al*. Renal angioplasty technical results and clinical outcome in 320 patients. *Mayo Clin Proc* 1995;70:1041–52

Derkx FHM, van Jaarsveld BC, Krijnen P, *et al*. Renal artery stenosis towards the year 2000. *J Hypertens* 1996;14(suppl 5):S167–72

Semple PF, Dominiczak AF. Detection and treatment of renovascular disease: 40 years on. *J Hypertens* 1994;12:729–34

Tegtmeyer CJ, Matsumoto AH, Angle JF. Percutaneous transluminal angioplasty in fibrous dysplasia. In Novick AC, ed. *Renal Vascular Disease*. London: WB Saunders, 1996:363–83

Renal hypertension

D'Amico G, Minetti L, Ponticelli C, *et al*. Prognostic indicators in idiopathic IgA mesangial nephropathy. *Quart J Med* 1986;59:363–78

Smith MC, Dunn MJ. Hypertension in renal parenchymal disease. In Laragh JH, Brenner BM, eds. *Hypertension: Pathophysiology, Diagnosis and Management*, 2nd edn. New York: Raven Press, 1996:2081–102

Diabetes mellitus

Böhlen L, De Courten M, Weidmann P. Comparative study of the effect of ACE inhibitors and other antihypertensives on proteinuria in diabetic patients. *Am J Hypertens* 1994;7(suppl 11):84S–92

Breyer JA. Medical management of nephropathy in type I diabetes mellitus: Current recommendations. *J Am Soc Nephrol* 1995;6:1523–9

Haffner SM, Ferrannini E, Hazudu HP, Stern MP. Clustering of cardiovascular risk factors in confirmed prehypertensive individuals. *Hypertension* 1992;20:38–45

Parving HH, Jacobsen P, Rossing K, *et al*. Benefits of long-term antihypertensive treatment in prognosis in diabetic nephropathy. *Kidney Int* 1996;49:1778–82

Reichard P, Nilsson B-Y, Rosenquist U. The effect of long-term intensified treatment in the development of microvascular complications of diabetes mellitus. *N Engl J Med* 1993;329:304–9

The Diabetes Control and Complications Trial Research Group. The effect of intensive treatment of diabetes on the development and progression of long-term complications in insulin-dependent diabetes mellitus. *N Engl J Med* 1993;329:977–86

Mineralocorticoid hypertension

Biglieri EG, Kater CE, Mantero F. Adrenocortical forms of human hypertension. In Laragh JH, Brenner BM, eds. *Hypertension: Pathophysiology, Diagnosis and Management,* 2nd edn. New York: Raven Press, 1996:2145–61

Semple PF. Mineralocorticoid excess. In James VHT, ed. *The Adrenal Gland,* 2nd edn. New York: Raven Press, 1992:373–89

Wharwood CB, Stewart PM. Human hypertension caused by mutation in the 11-hydroxysteroid dehydrogenase gene: A molecular analysis of apparent mineralocorticoid excess. *J Hypertens* 1996;14(suppl 5):S19–24

Whitworth JA. Mechanisms of glucocorticoid-induced hypertension. *Kidney Int* 1987;31:1213–24

Pheochromocytoma

Manger WM, Gifford RW. Pheochromocytoma: A clinical overview. Adrenocortical forms of human hypertension. In Laragh JH, Brenner BM, eds. *Hypertension: Pathophysiology, Diagnosis and Management,* 2nd edn. New York: Raven Press, 1996:2225–44

Hyperparathyroidism

Dominiczak AF, Lyall F, Morton JJ, *et al.* Blood pressure, left ventricular mass and intracellular calcium in primary hyperparathyroidism. *Clin Sci* 1990;78:127–32

Coarctation of the aorta

Hougen TJ, Sell JE. Recent advances in the diagnosis and treatment of coarctation of the aorta. *Curr Opin Cardiol* 1995;10:524–9

Interactions with lipids

Pederson TR. Primary prevention of cardiovascular disease. *J Hypertens* 1996;14 (suppl 5):S195–200

Sacks FM, Pfeffer MA, Moye LA, *et al.* The effect of pravastatin on coronary events after myocardial infarction in patients with average cholesterol levels. *N Engl J Med* 1996;335:1001–9

Scandinavian Simvastatin Survival Study (4S). Randomized trial of cholesterol-lowering in 4444 patients with coronary heart disease. *Lancet* 1994; 344:1383–9

Shepherd J, Cobbe SM, Ford I, *et al.* Prevention of coronary heart disease with pravastatin in men with hypercholesterolemia. *N Engl J Med* 1995; 333:1301–7

General

Laragh JH, Brenner BM, eds. *Hypertension,* vols I & II, 2nd edn. New York: Raven Press, 1995

Swales J, ed. *Textbook of Hypertension.* London: Blackwell Scientific Publishers, 1994

Section 2 Hypertension Illustrated

List of illustrations

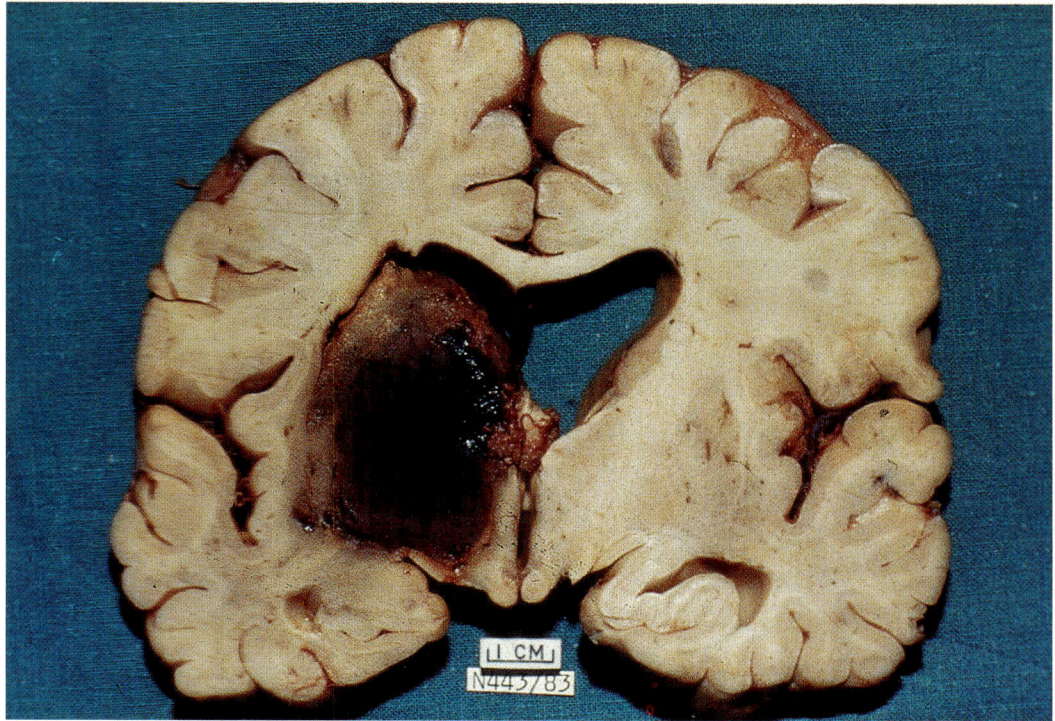

Figure 1 Coronal section of brain showing hemorrhage in the putamen of a patient with hypertension. Bleeding originates from 'miliary' aneurysms in short perforating arteries, as proposed by Charcot and Bouchard in 1889

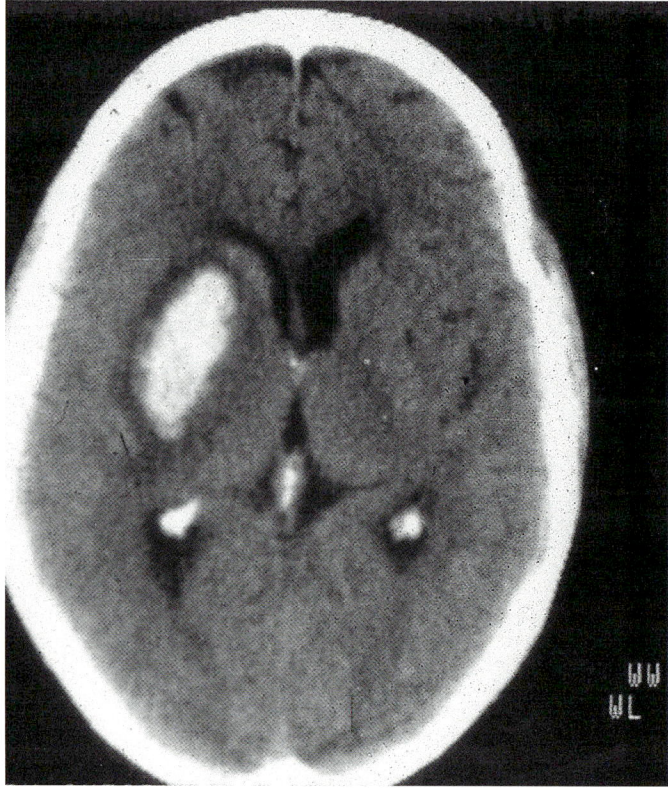

Figure 2 Computed tomography (CT) shows hemorrhage into the right putamen in a patient with uncontrolled hypertension. There was severe hemiplegia and hemianesthesia with visuospatial neglect

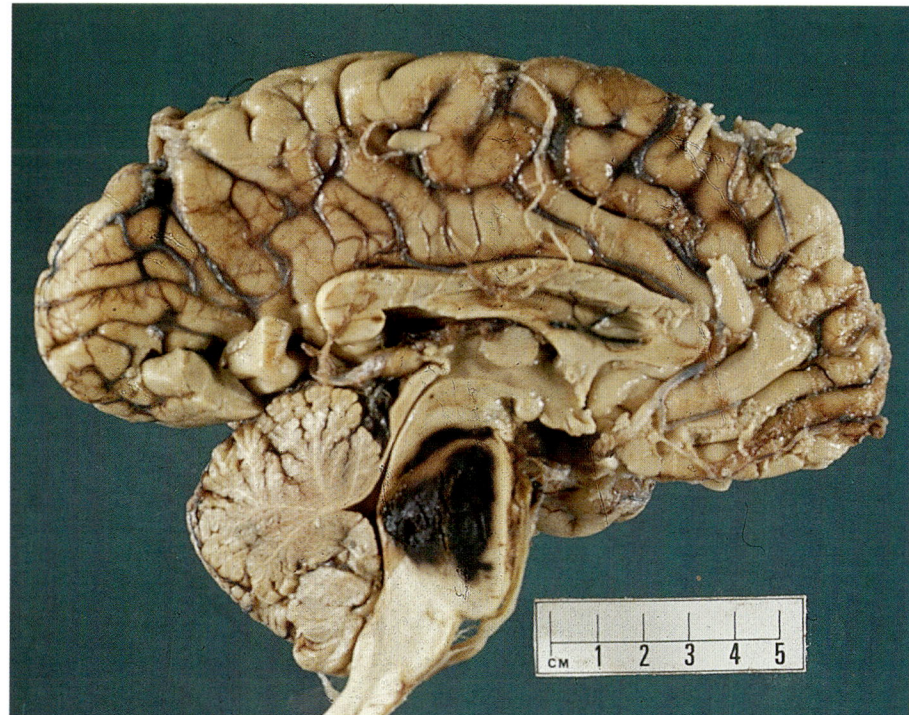

Figure 3 Sagittal section of brain showing hemorrhage in the pons, which comprises around 5% of all hypertensive intracerebral hemorrhages. Most of these hemorrhages cause early coma and are fatal

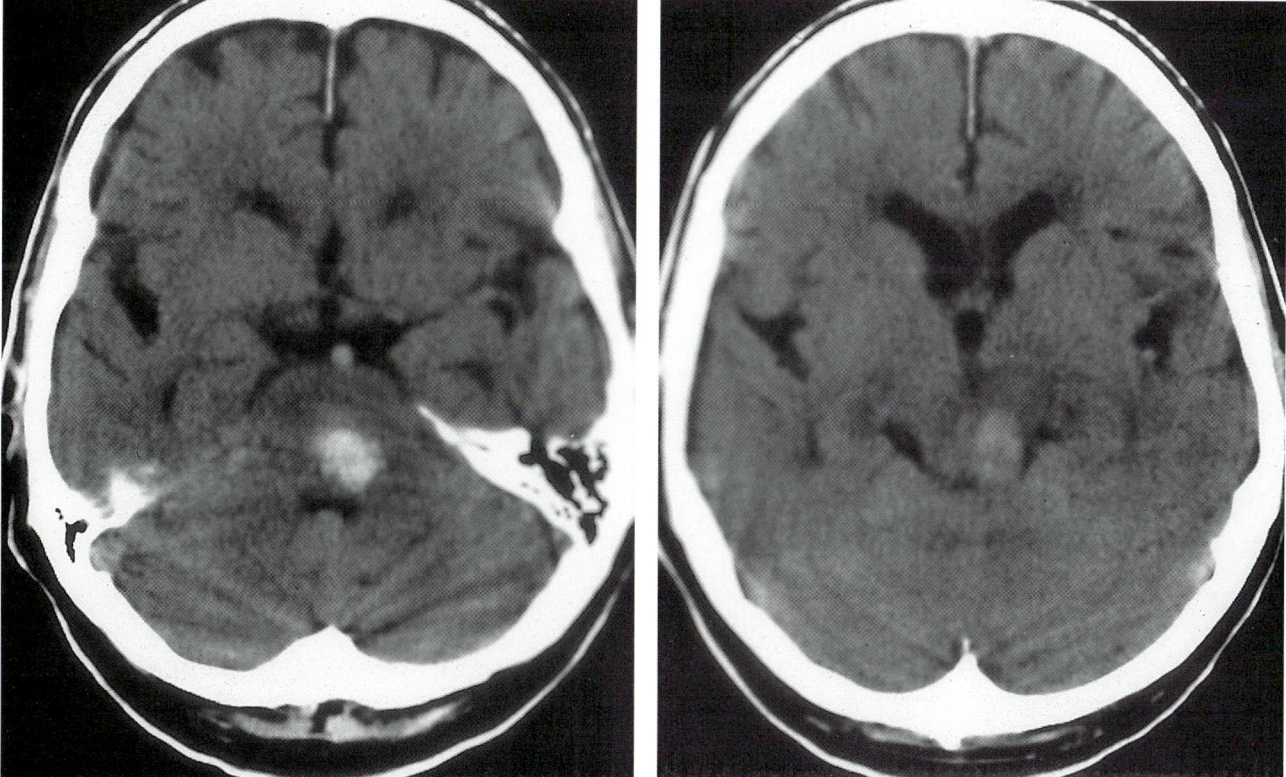

Figure 4 CTs showing hypertensive hemorrhage into the tegmentum pontis (left) which extends up into the midbrain (right). There was bilateral gaze palsy with ocular bobbing and ataxic right hemiparesis

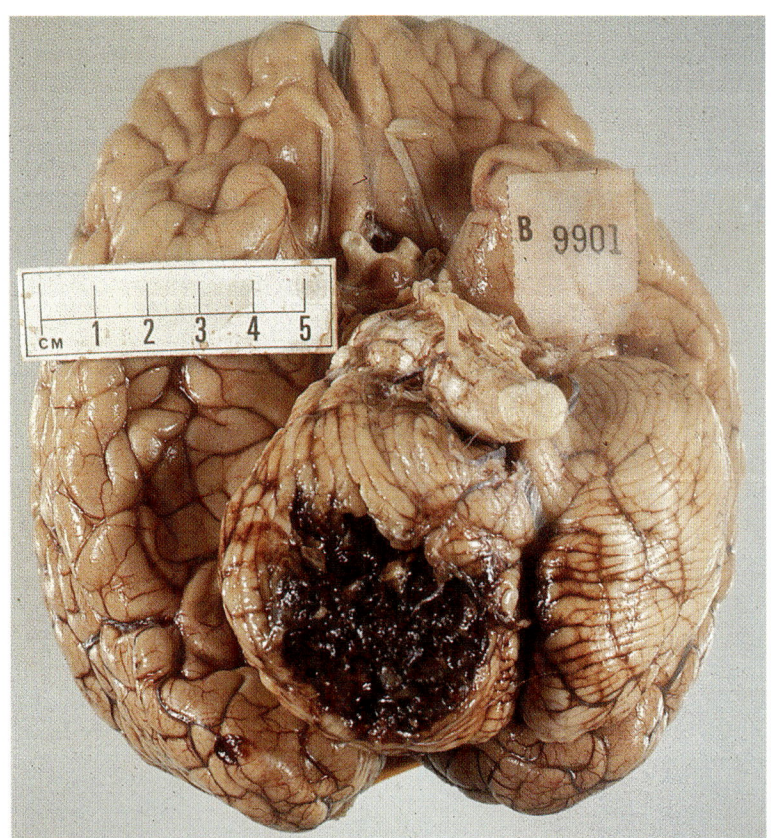

Figure 5 Brain viewed from the base showing another consequence of hypertension, hemorrhage into the cerebellum. Common presenting symptoms are occipital headache, vomiting, vertigo and an inability to stand

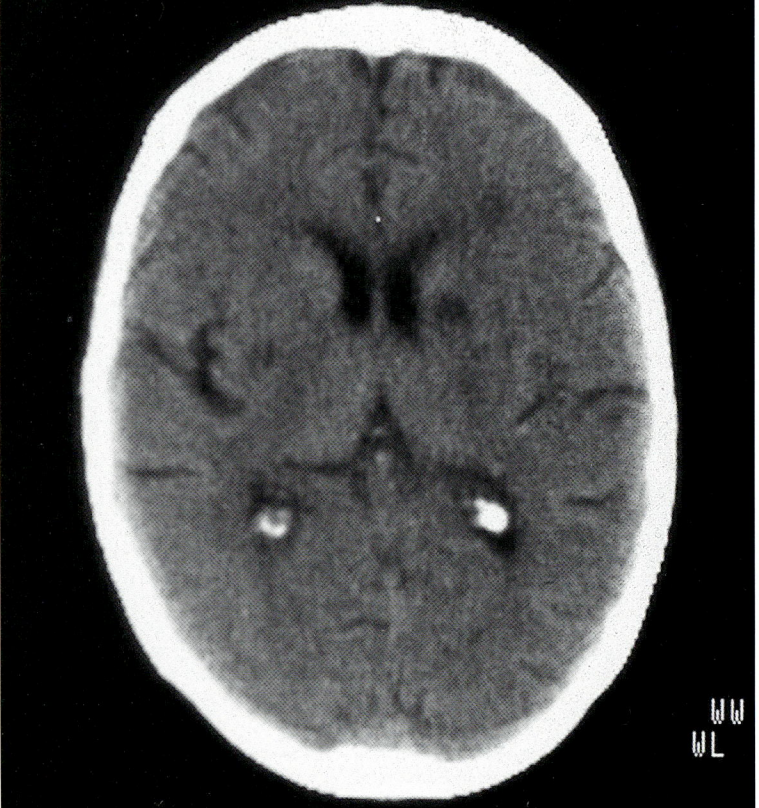

Figure 6 CT showing lacunar infarction in poorly controlled hypertension. The small infarct abutting on the caudate nucleus is very well-defined. Infarcts of this type are the result of occlusion of penetrating end arteries and are often too small to be seen on CT. Pure motor hemiparesis is a typical lacunar syndrome resulting from infarction in the internal capsule or basis pontis

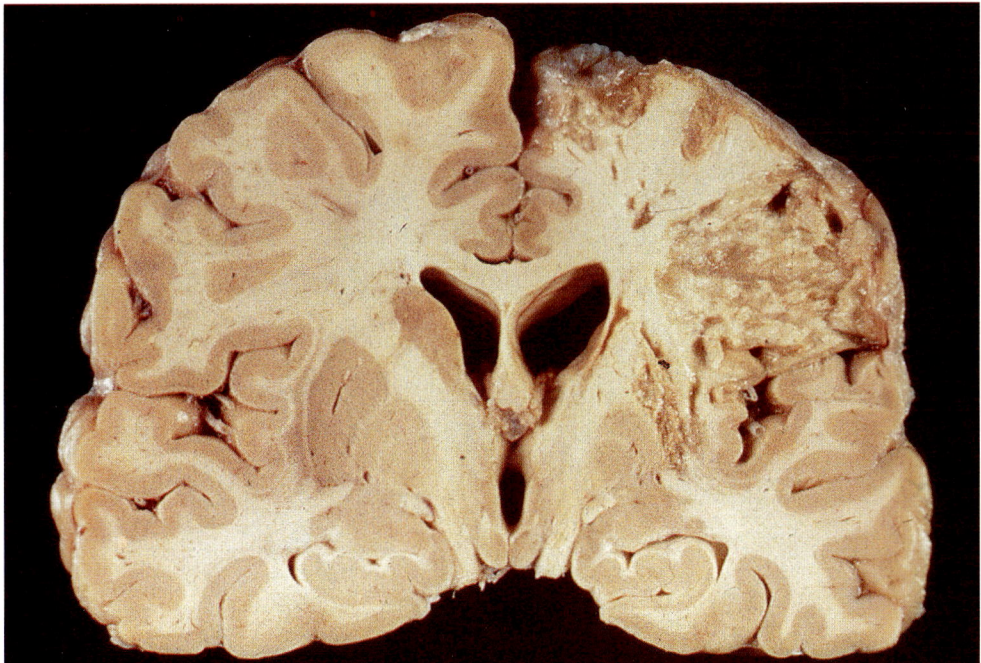

Figure 7 Coronal section of brain showing an established infarct in the distribution of the middle cerebral artery. Infarction in this territory is often the result of occlusion in the extracranial internal carotid artery

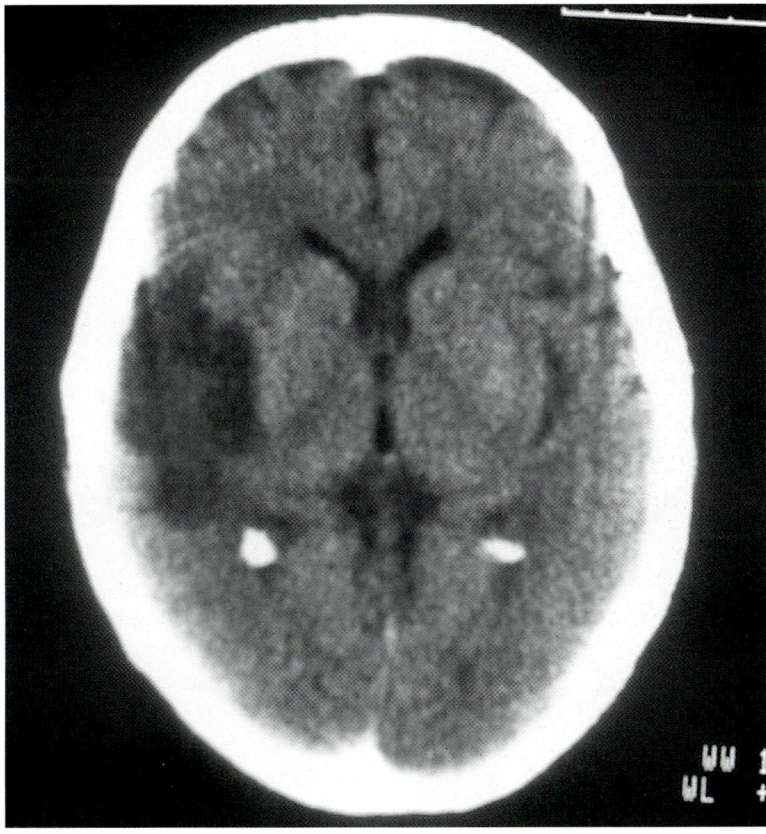

Figure 8 CT showing a well-defined old infarct in the superficial territory of the middle cerebral artery

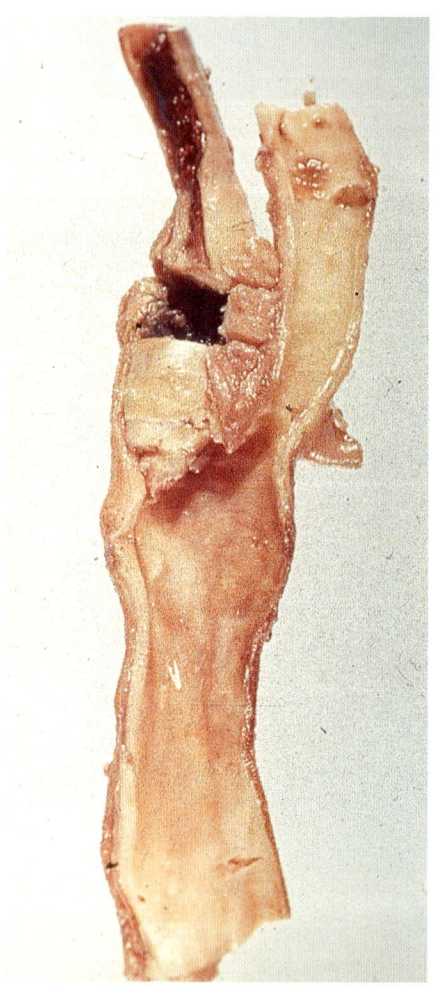
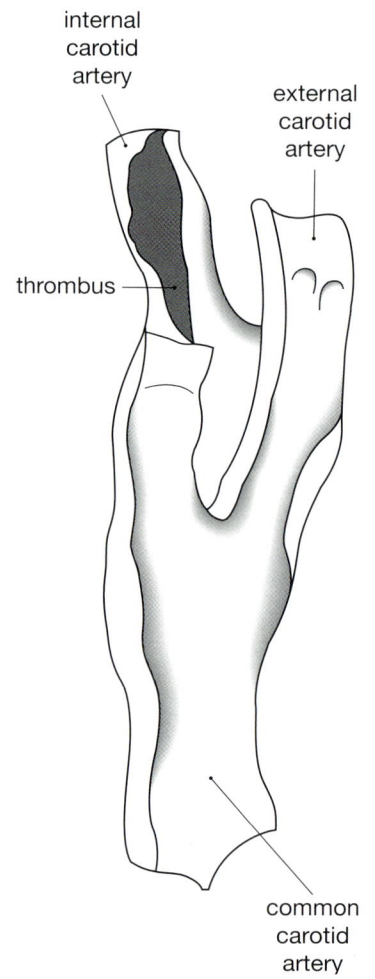

internal
carotid
artery

external
carotid
artery

thrombus

common
carotid
artery

Figure 9 Postmortem section of the carotid artery at the bifurcation showing considerable atheroma in the internal carotid artery. The artery is occluded by thrombus

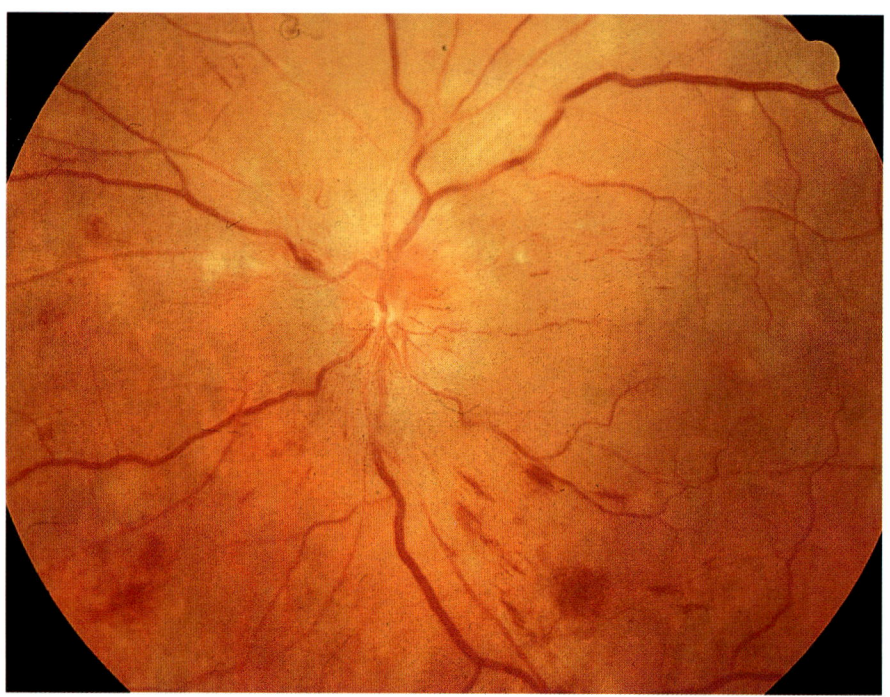

Figure 10 Funduscopy of a patient with malignant hypertension showing linear or flame-shaped retinal hemorrhages and papilledema. For a clinical diagnosis of malignant hypertension, such hemorrhages must be present in both eyes

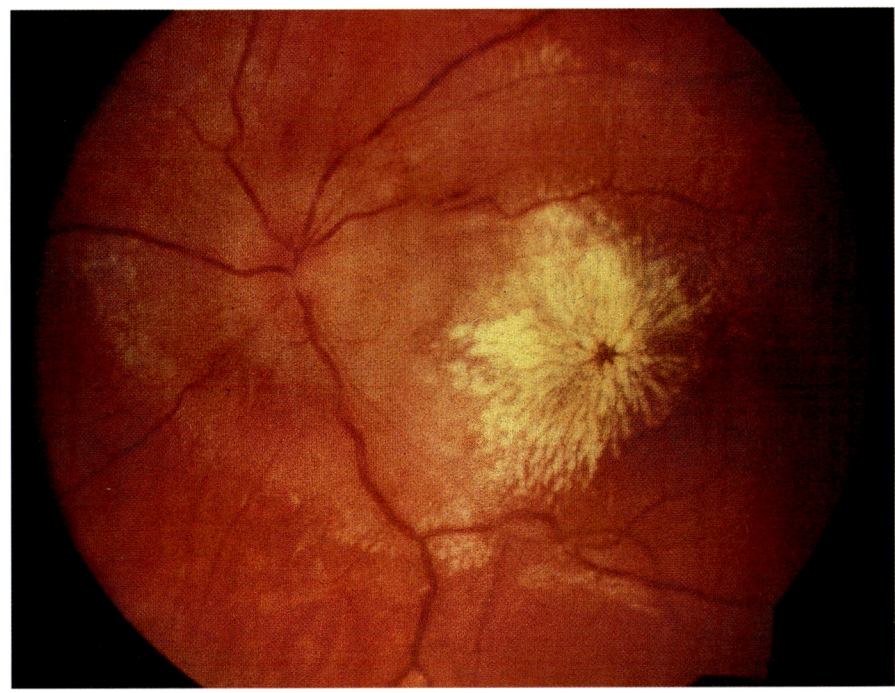

Figure 11 Funduscopy of a patient with malignant hypertension showing papilledema and prominent hard exudates; these exudates are referred to as a macular star

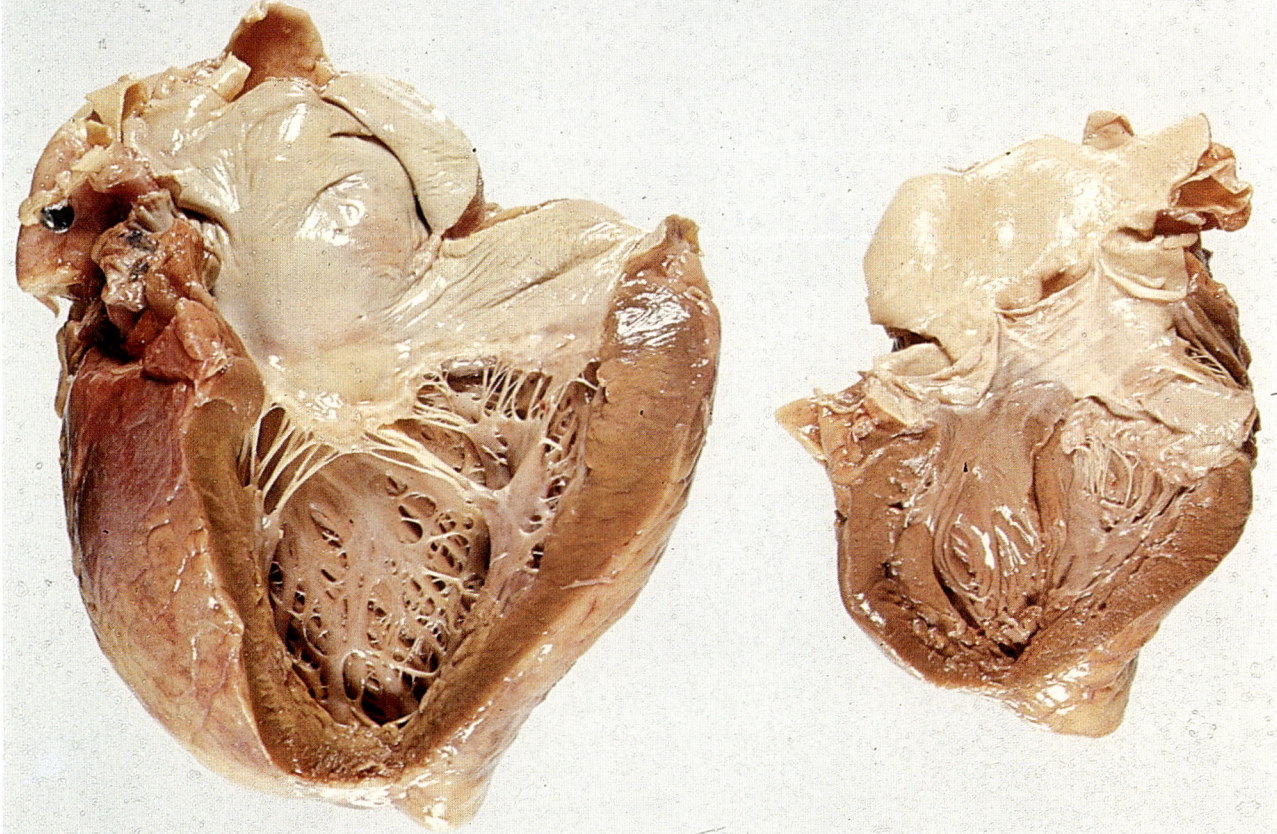

Figure 12 Coronal sections of a heart from a patient who had high blood pressure (left) compared with a normal heart (right). Note the increase in the overall size of the hypertensive heart and in the thickness of the left ventricular wall

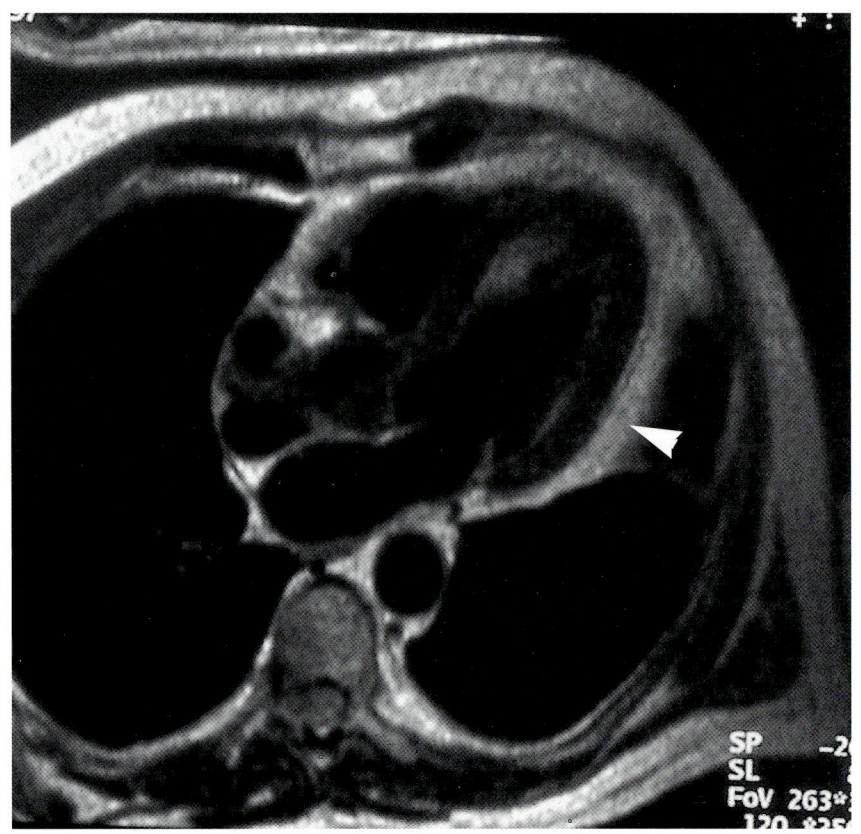

Figure 13 MRI (long-axis view) of left ventricular hypertrophy (LVH; left ventricle is arrowed) in a middle-aged patient with resistant hypertension. The hypertrophy is concentric and the leaflets of the mitral valve can be clearly seen below and to the left. MRI is probably superior to echocardiography in quantifying ventricular hypertrophy

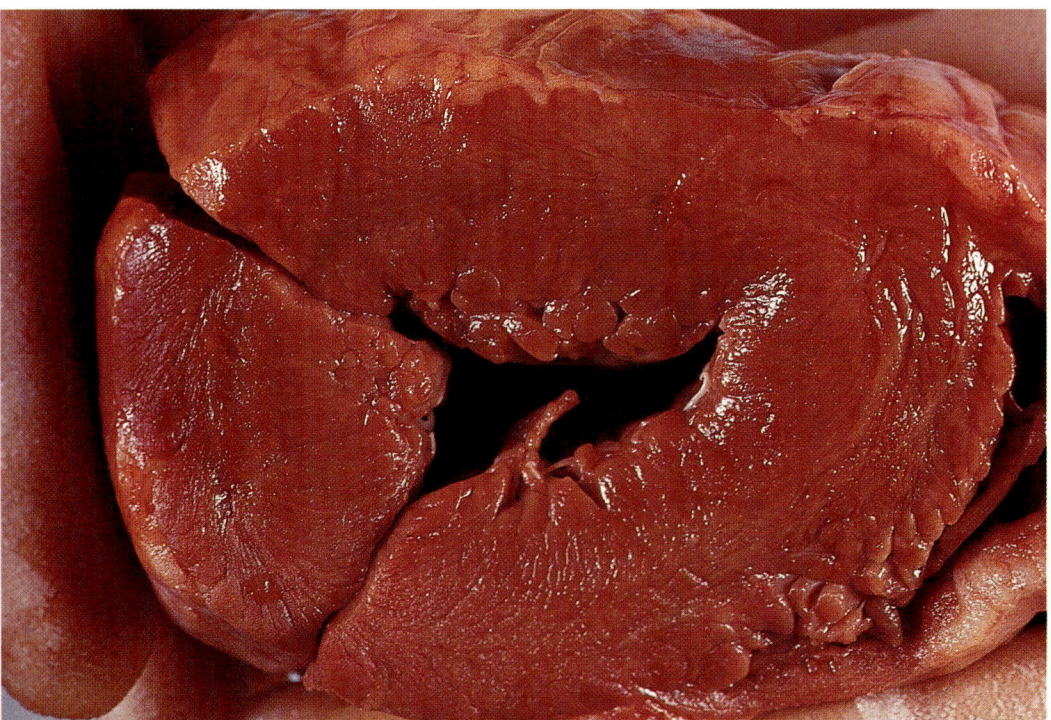

Figure 14 Transverse section of a heart in chronic severe hypertension shows marked LVH

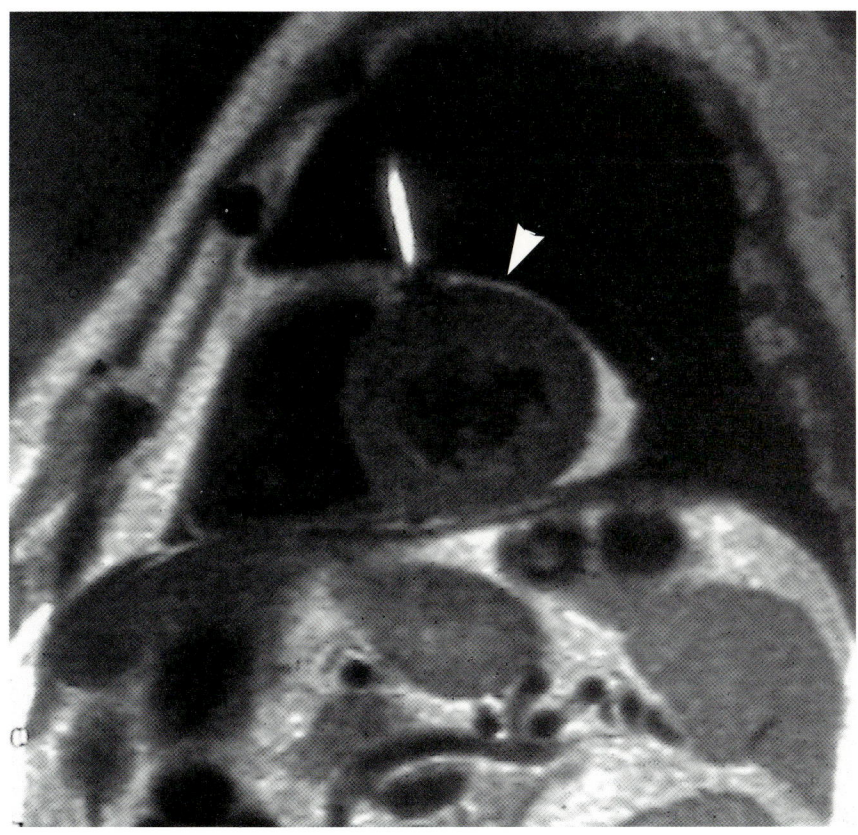

Figure 15 MRI (short-axis view) of the same patient as in Figure 13 showing concentric LVH (arrowed)

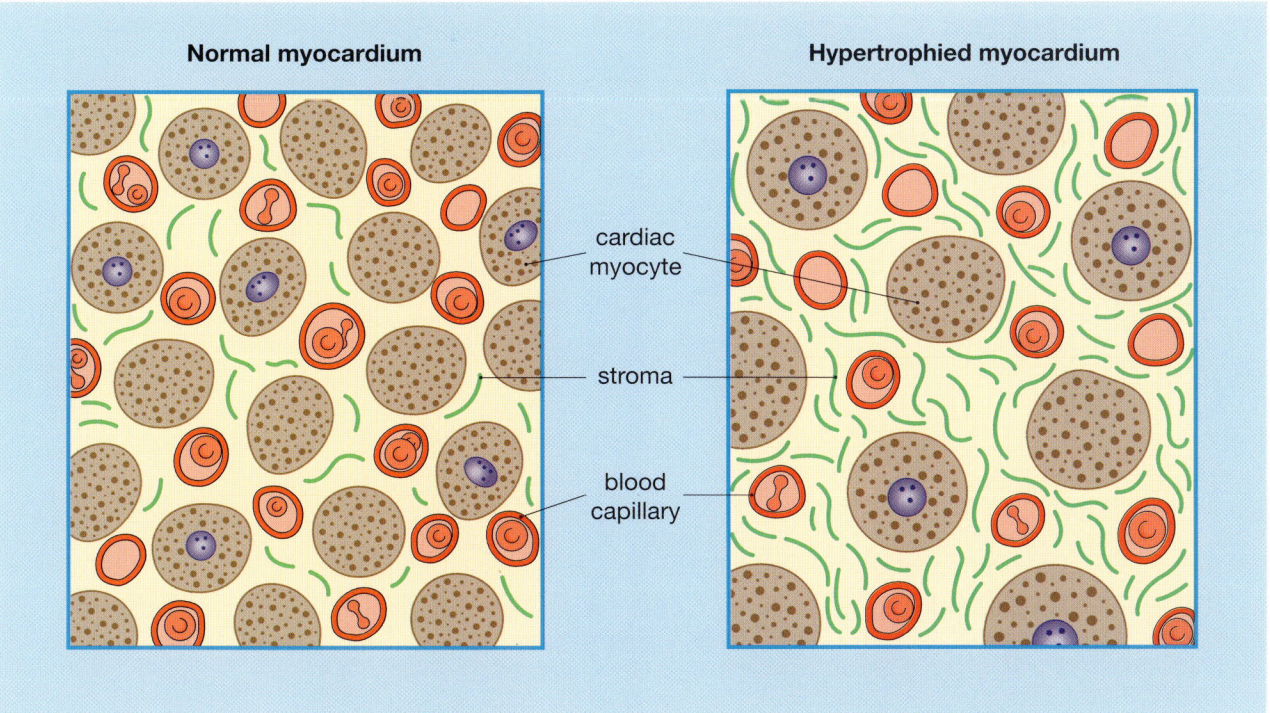

Figure 16 Schematic diagrams showing the typical appearances of normal (left) compared with hypertrophied (right) myocardium

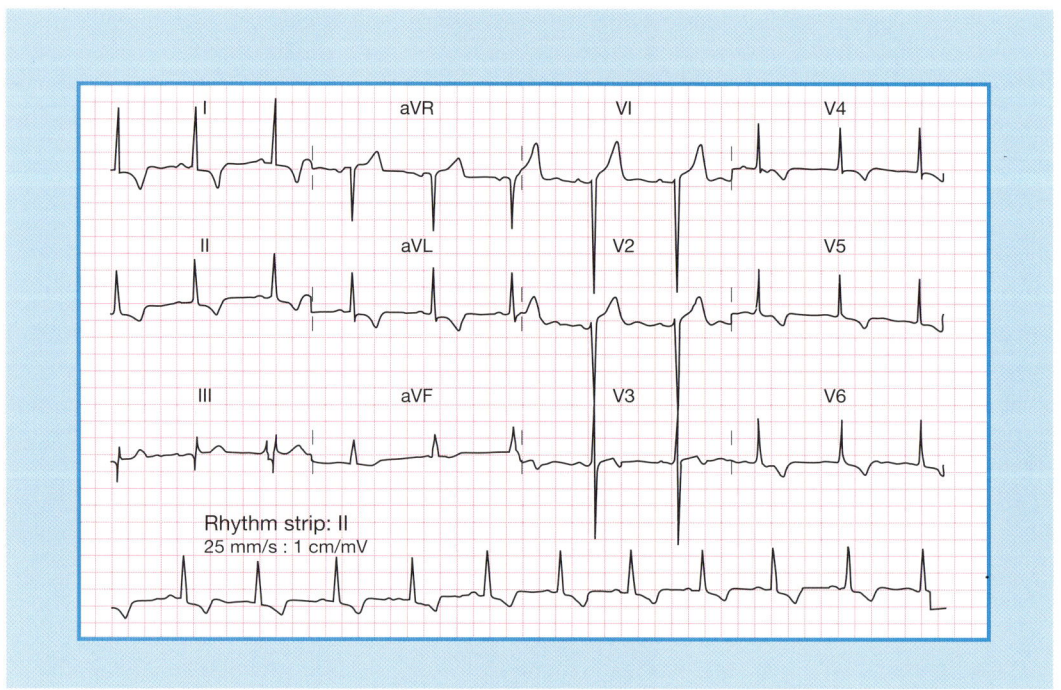

Figure 17 ECG in severe hypertension shows evidence of LVH by limb- and chest-lead voltage criteria. There is ST-segment depression in the lateral leads, described as the 'strain' pattern. The usual chest-lead criterion for LVH is: S wave in V1 + R wave in V5 > 35 mm. Criteria in limb leads are: R wave in V1 + S wave in V3 > 25 mm or R wave in lead 1 > 12 mm

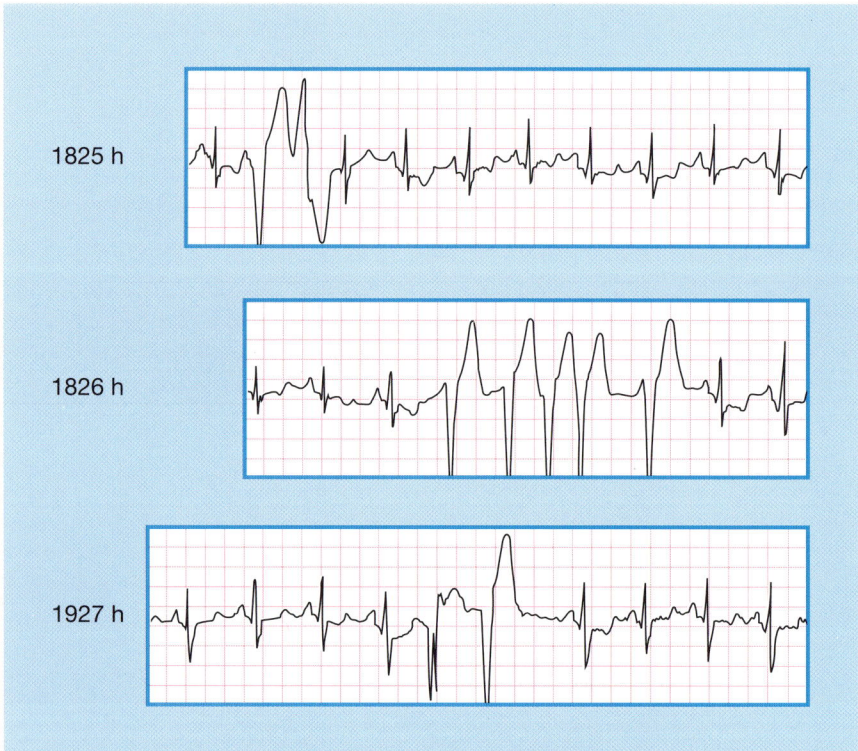

Figure 18 Extracts from a 24-h ECG of a patient with LVH due to hypertension shows a short burst of ventricular tachycardia (middle section). Ventricular hypertrophy in hypertension may be an independent risk factor for cardiovascular events. In treated hypertensive patients, there is an association among hypertrophy, ventricular arrhythmias and sudden death

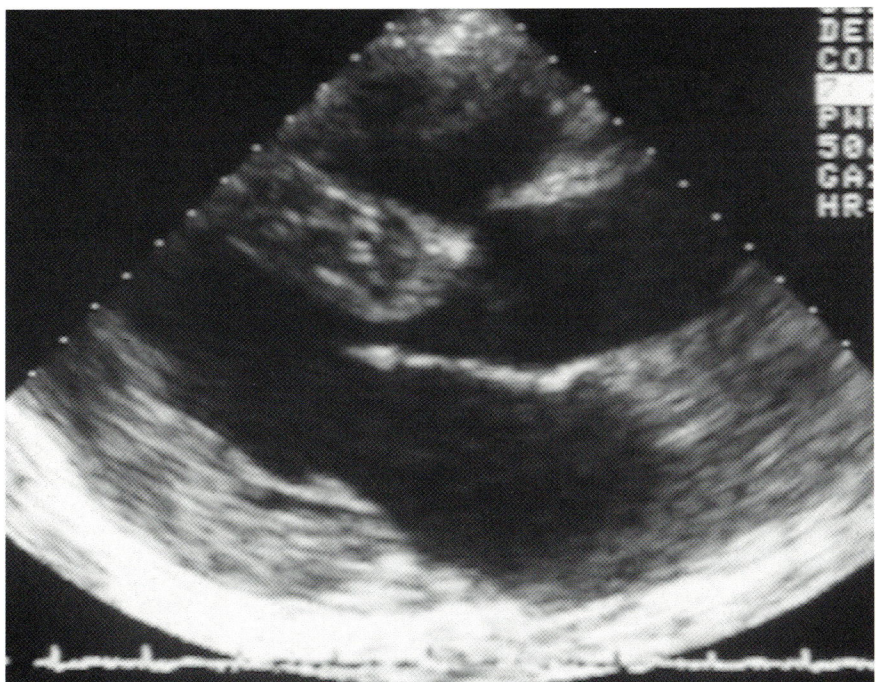

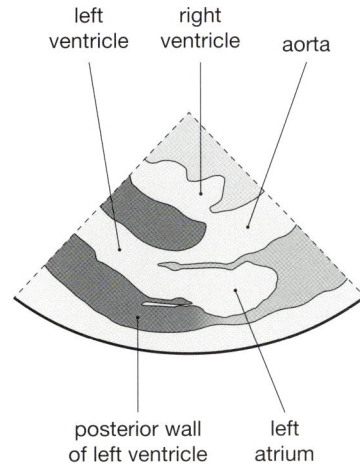

left ventricle   right ventricle   aorta

posterior wall of left ventricle   left atrium

Figure 19 Two-dimensional (2-D) echocardiogram (long-axis view) showing concentric LVH with increased thickness of both the interventricular septum and the posterior wall (normal thickness is ≤ 12 mm). The aorta is somewhat dilated as a result of stretching of the walls due to arteriosclerosis. Echocardiography is more sensitive than ECG in detecting LVH in hypertension

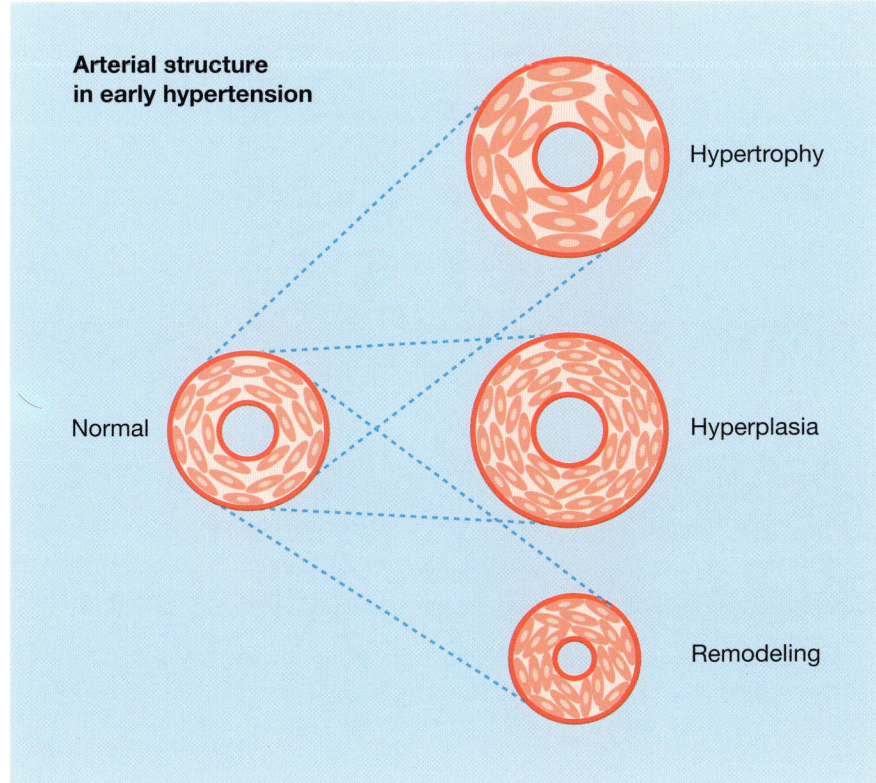

Arterial structure in early hypertension

Hypertrophy

Normal

Hyperplasia

Remodeling

Figure 20 Schematic diagram showing three types of thickening of the media in resistance arterioles caused by hypertension. Such thickening results in an increase in wall: lumen ratio

51

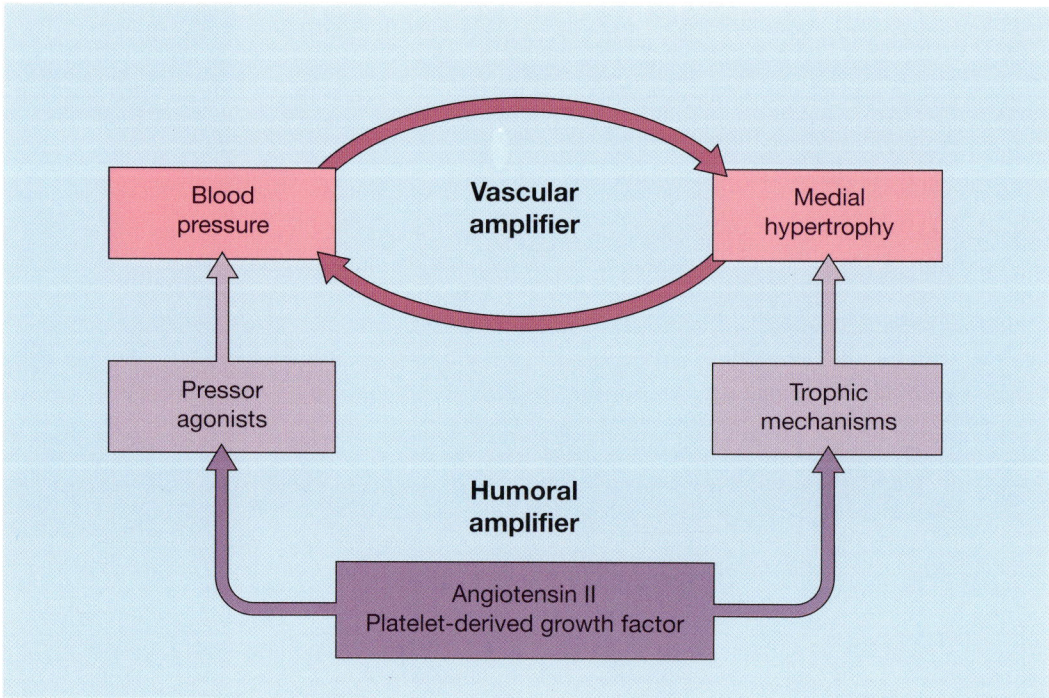

Figure 21 Schematic diagram of the humoral amplifier showing the pathways by which local and circulating vasoconstrictors may also promote medial hypertrophy

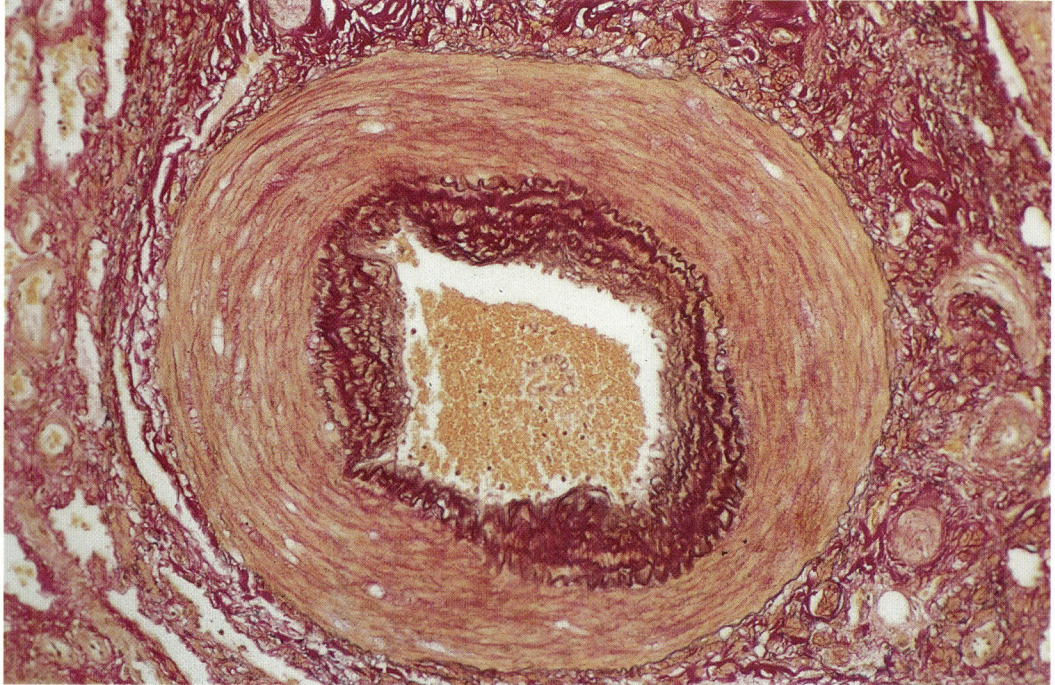

Figure 22 Histology showing a renal artery in the early stages of established hypertension showing medial hypertrophy and intimal thickening causing an increase in wall:lumen ratio. Intimal thickening is a result of an increase in collagen and elastic (black-staining) matrix proteins (elastica van Gieson)

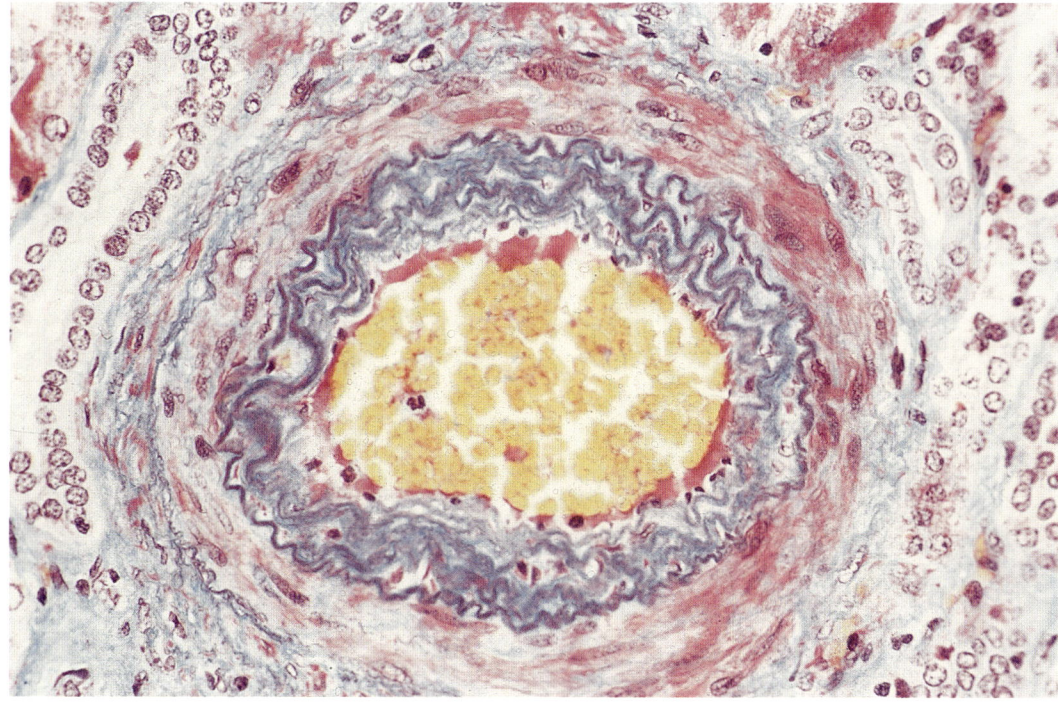

Figure 23 Histology showing a renal artery with thickening of the intima due to reduplication of the internal elastic lamina (blue-staining). The media is now thinner because of smooth muscle cell atrophy (elastica Martius scarlet–blue)

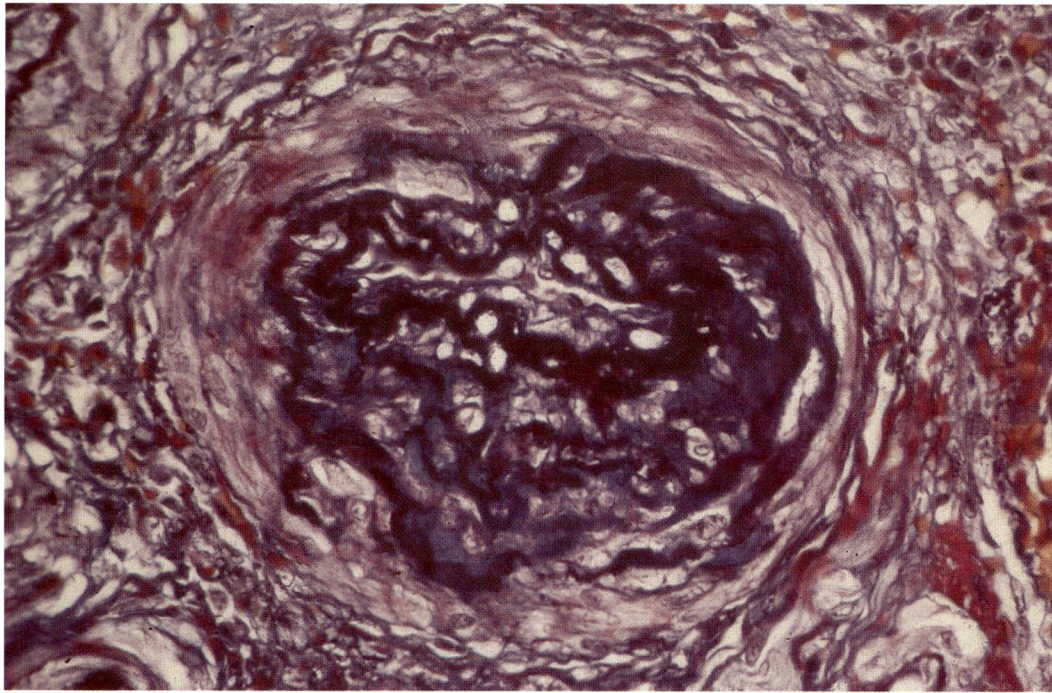

Figure 24 Histology showing a renal artery with severe arteriosclerosis such that most of the artery comprises a thickened intima with prominent reduplication of the internal elastic lamina. The media is atrophic and contains little smooth muscle (elastica Martius scarlet–blue)

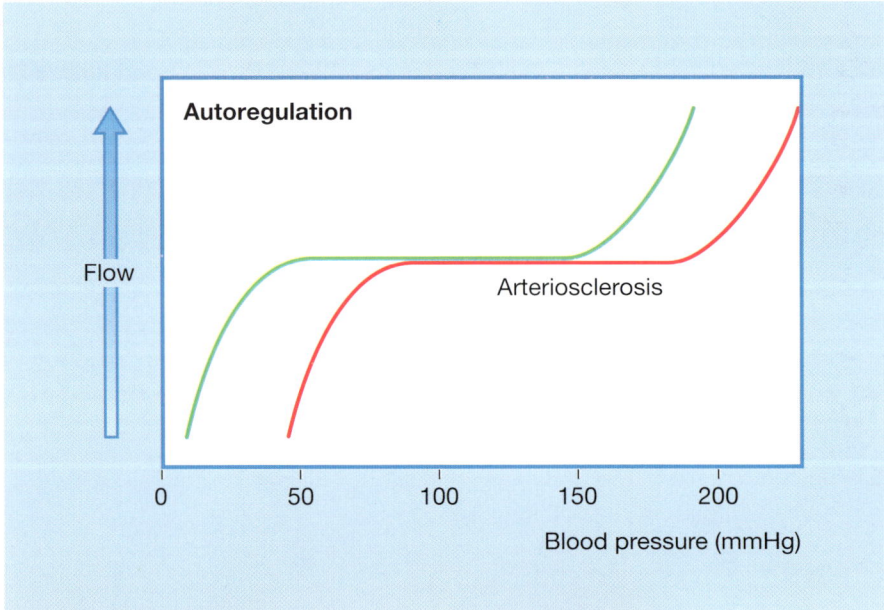

Figure 25 In the cerebral and renal circulations, autoregulation maintains constant blood flow over a range of pressures. Arteriosclerosis due to hypertension or aging causes a shift of the autoregulatory curve to the right. As a consequence, the risk of cerebral and renal underperfusion during hypotension is increased, although susceptibility to malignant-phase hypertension is reduced

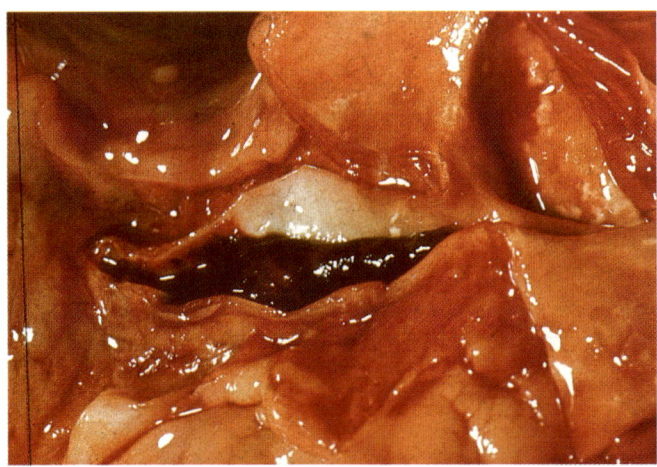

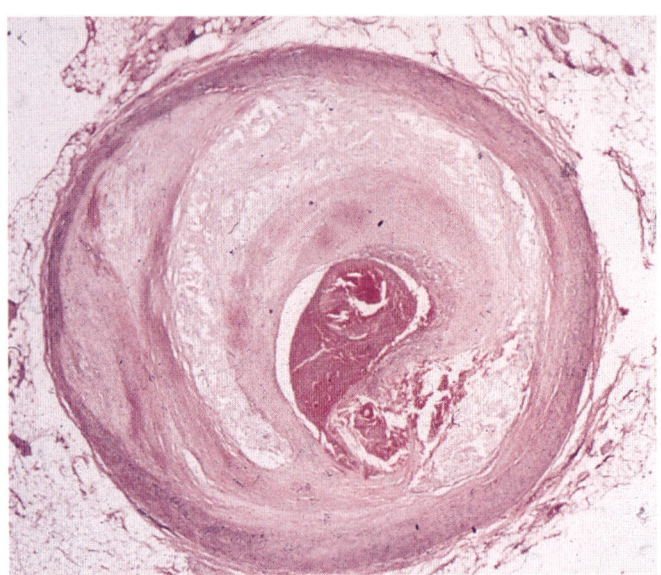

Figure 26 Recent thrombus (arrowed) can be seen at the origin of the right coronary artery close to the aorta (upper). Histology showing a severely atheromatous coronary artery (lower) shows residual media (deep pink-staining). The artery is narrowed by atheromatous plaque comprising a mixture of pale fibrous tissue and clear lipid material. The plaque cap has ruptured, causing hemorrhage into the plaque and thrombosis of the lumen (H & E)

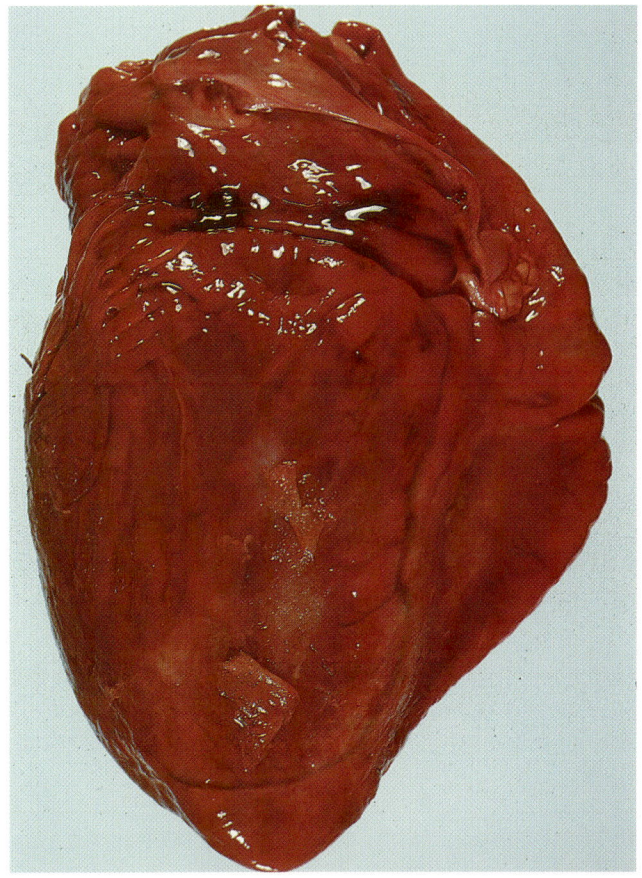

Figure 27 Postmortem heart 7 days after anterior myocardial infarction. Note the roughening of the epicardium due to pericarditis

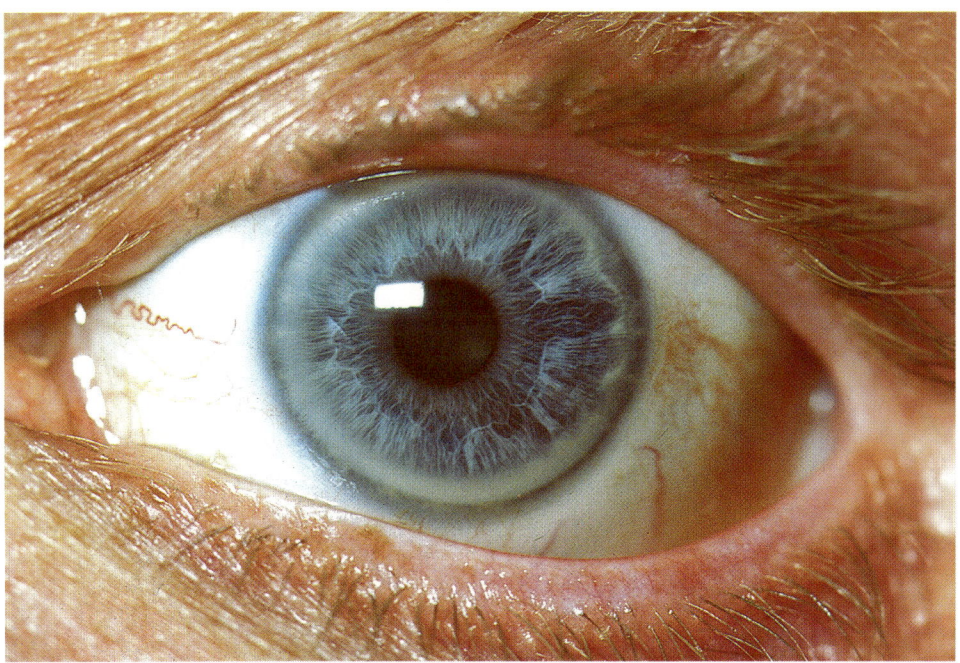

Figure 28 Eye showing a corneal arcus. Such a development before the age of 60 years often signifies hypercholesterolemia and is associated with a high risk of coronary artery disease

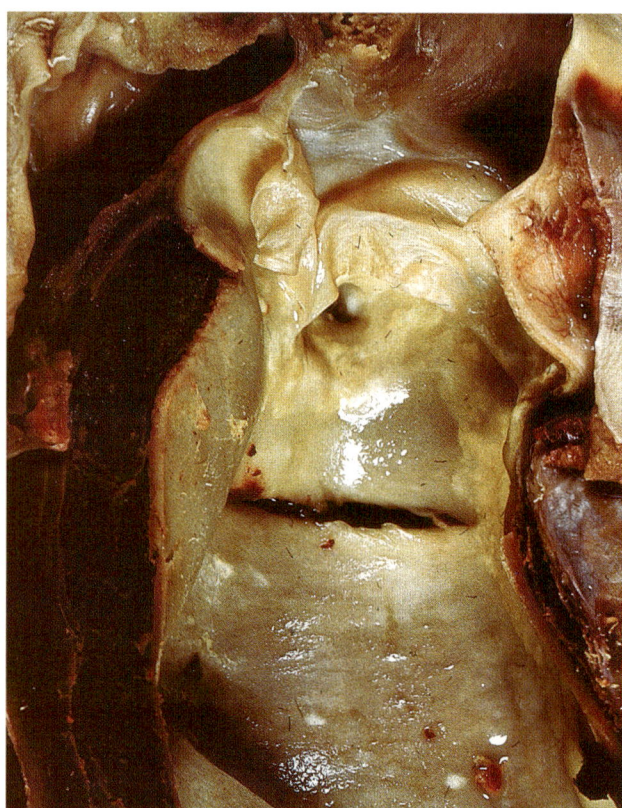

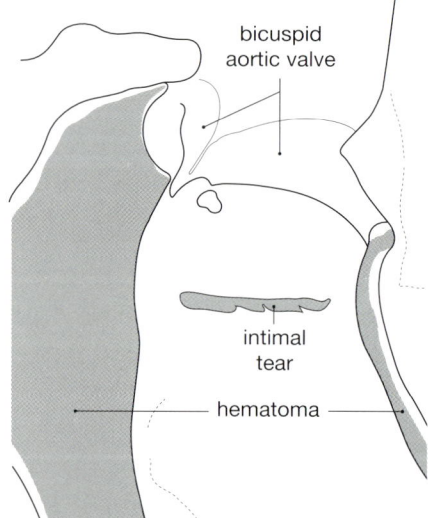

Figure 29 Aorta showing a typical transverse tear (2.5 cm) on the inner aspect around 3 cm above the aortic valve, the site of initiation of around 60% of cases of aortic dissection. Hematoma can be seen on the inner surface of the vessel. Hypertension is the most common factor predisposing to aortic dissection

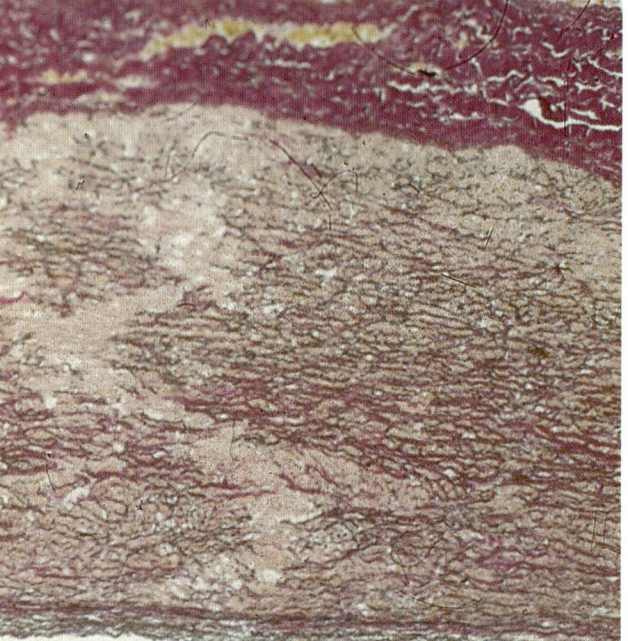

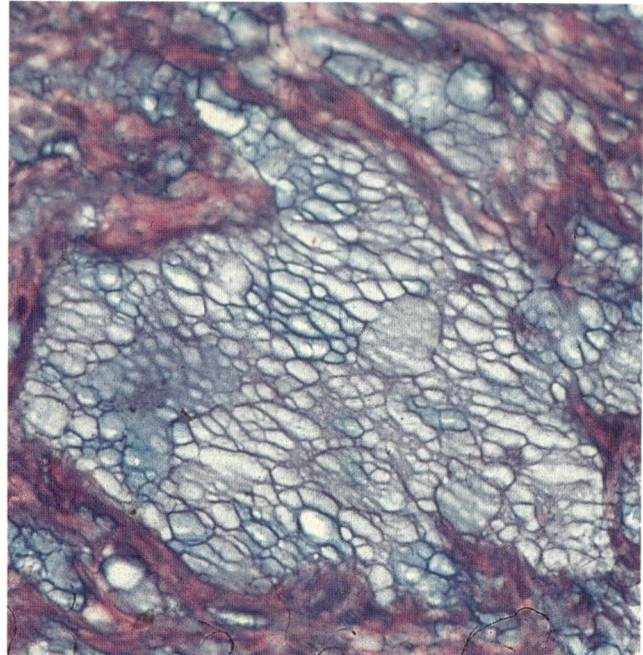

Figure 30 Histology of the aorta in a case of fatal aortic dissection. Low power shows magenta-staining collagen and black-staining fragments of elastic laminae in the media with patchy loss of elastic tissue and smooth muscle (left). High power shows that the spaces in the media are, in fact, 'lakes' of proteoglycans (right) [periodic acid–Schiff (PAS)–alcian blue]

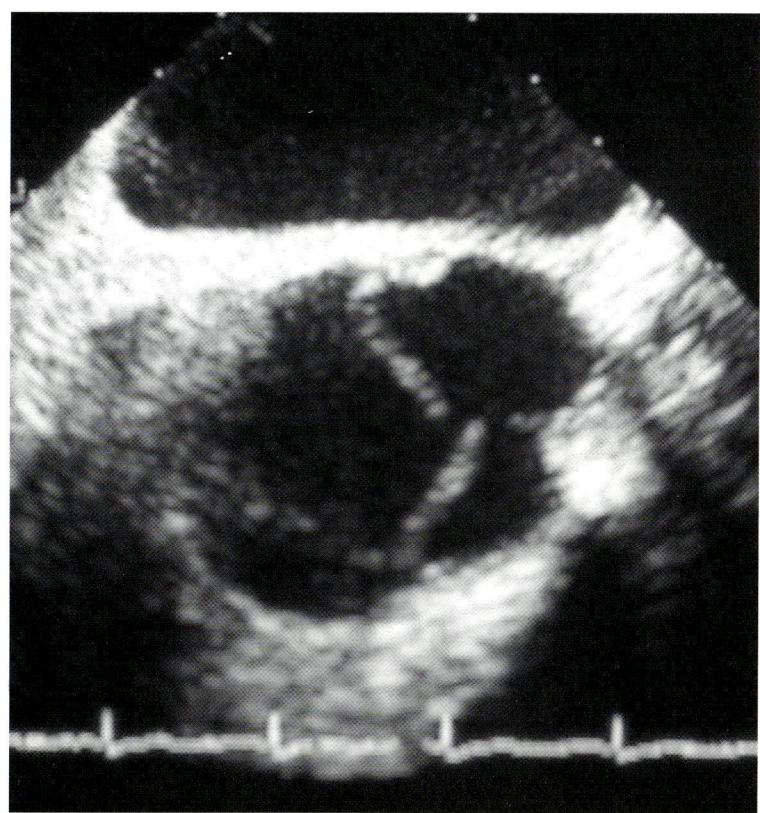

Figure 31 Transesophageal 2-D echocardiogram of the aorta showing a flap and tear, and a false lumen which probably contains thrombus. Color Doppler imaging (CDI) showed lower flow velocities in the false, compared with true, lumen

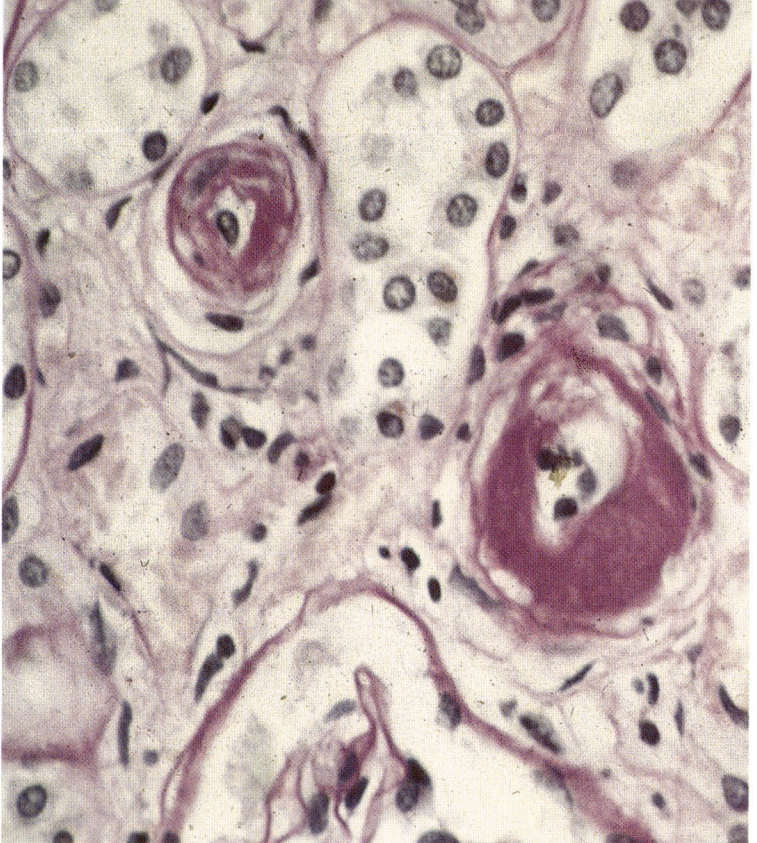

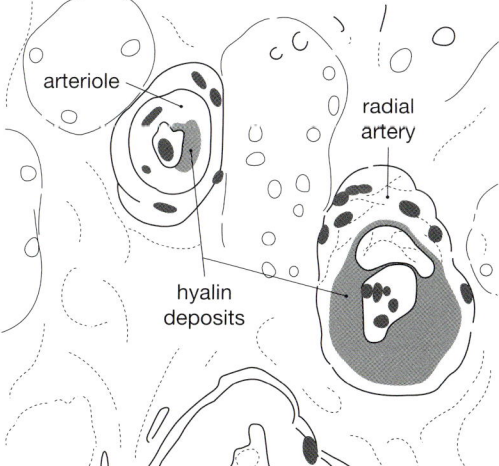

Figure 32 Histology showing arteriolosclerosis in a small renal artery and arteriole. The medial smooth muscle cells have been replaced by deposits of glycoprotein, comprising both protein derived from plasma and synthesized matrix protein, leading to wall thickening and luminal narrowing of the small arteries and arterioles in chronic hypertension (elastica Martius scarlet–blue)

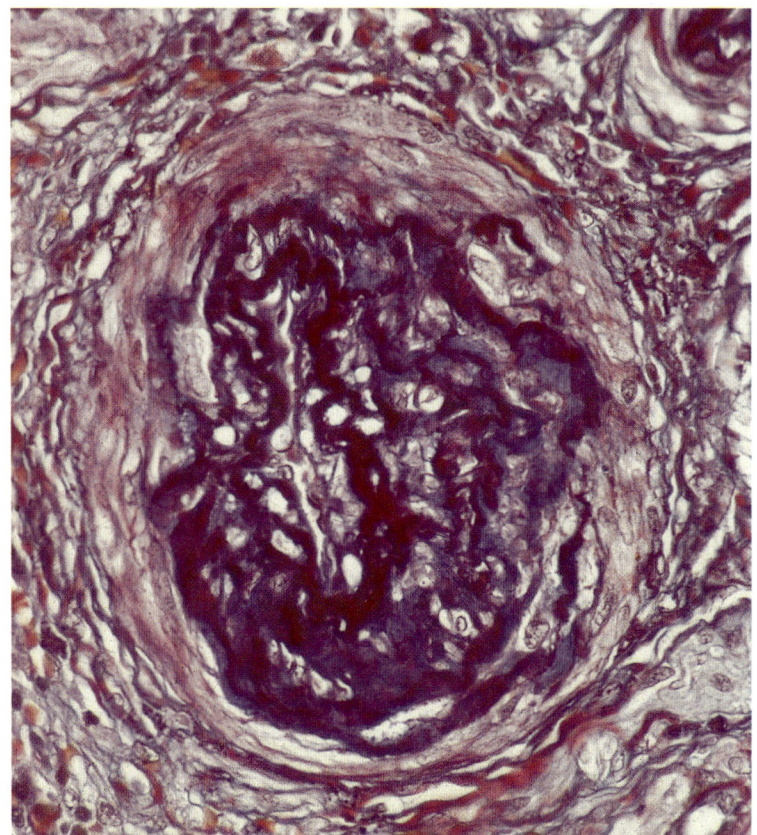

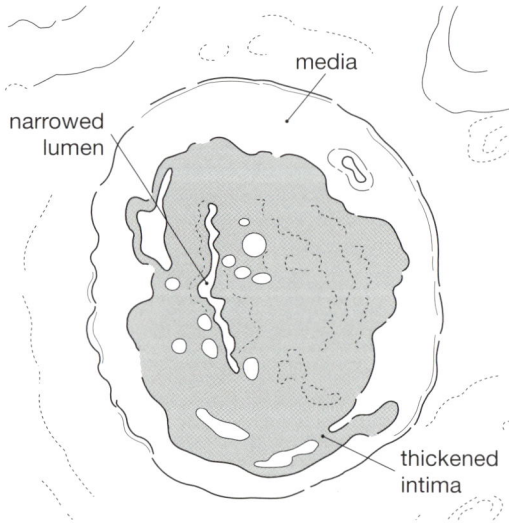

Figure 33 Histology showing an inter-lobular renal artery with arteriosclerosis and stained to reveal elastic tissue. There is considerable intimal thickening due to fibrosis with reduplication of the internal elastic lamina and atrophy of the media. Similar changes occur in old age (PAS)

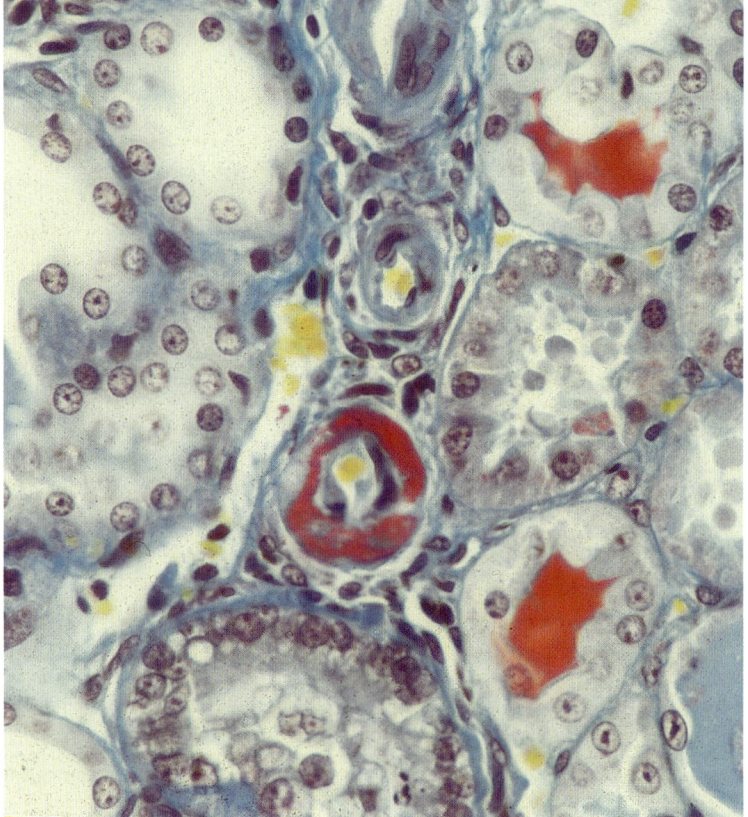

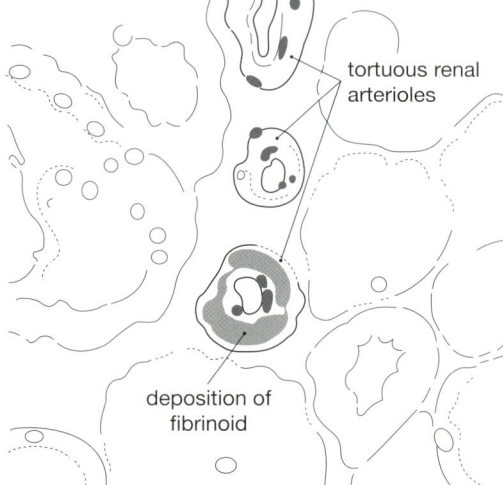

Figure 34 Histology of a kidney in severe hypertension showing red-staining 'fibri-noid' deposition in the media of an arteriole, a result of insudation of plasma proteins such as fibrinogen and fibrin. Proteins gain entry because vascular permeability is increased in response to damage caused by high intraluminal pressures (Martius scarlet–blue)

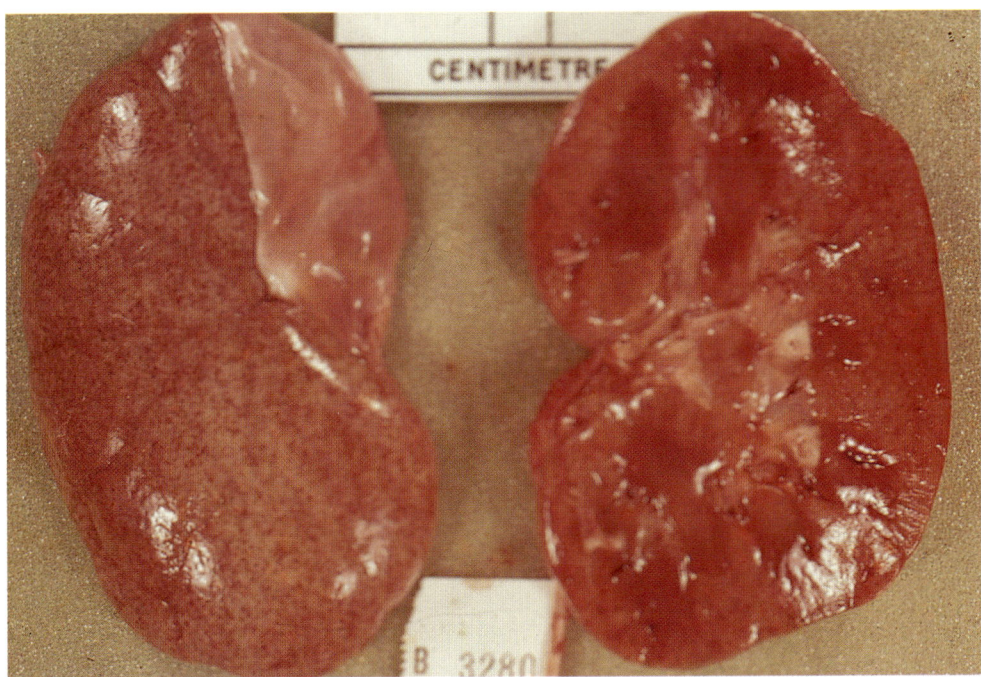

Figure 35 Kidneys in malignant-phase hypertension are swollen and edematous. The renal capsule has been removed to show the tiny punctate hemorrhages on the surface characteristic of the so-called 'flea-bitten' kidney

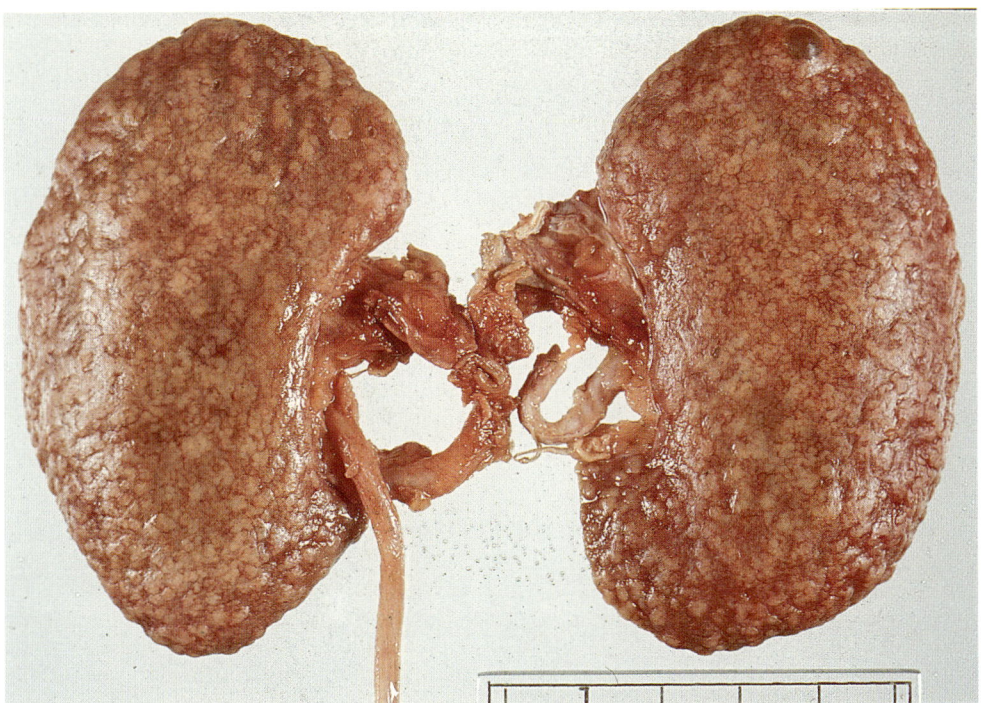

Figure 36 Kidneys from a patient who died several years after treatment for malignant hypertension show a granular surface due to ischemic scarring caused by proliferative endarteritis in the healing phase of severe hypertension

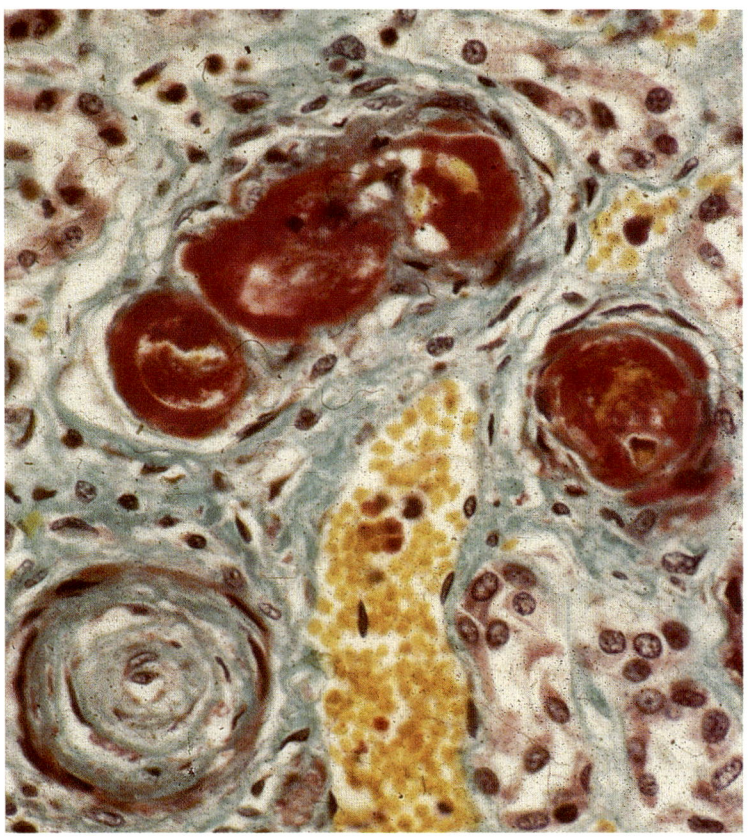

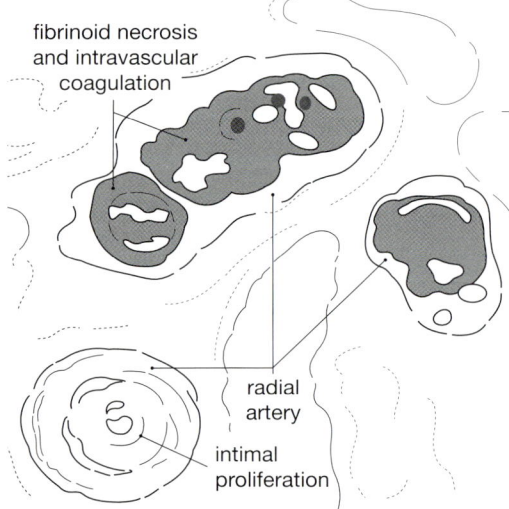

Figure 37 Histology of kidney in malignant hypertension showing areas of fibrinoid necrosis and intravascular coagulation. The remaining terminal interlobular artery shows 'onion-skin' proliferative endarteritis probably as a healing response to acute injury (Masson trichrome)

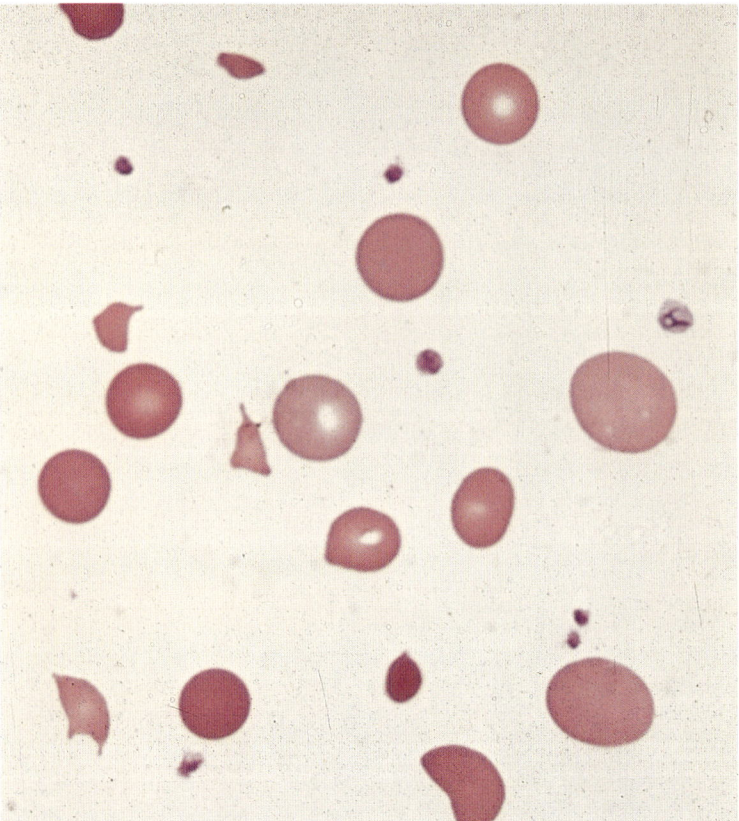

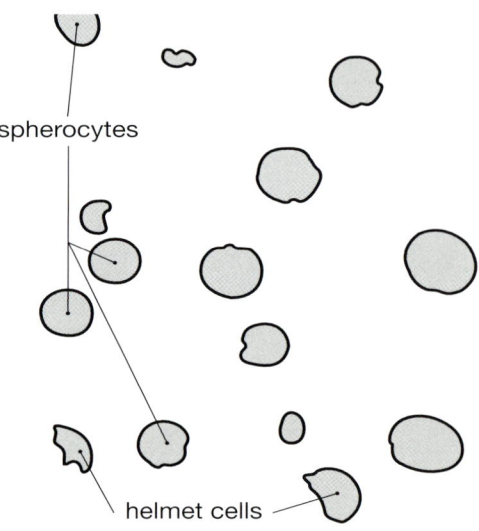

Figure 38 Blood film in malignant or accelerated hypertension may sometimes show red-cell fragmentation, and helmet cells and spherocytes typical of microangiopathic hemolytic anemia. The platelet count is usually low

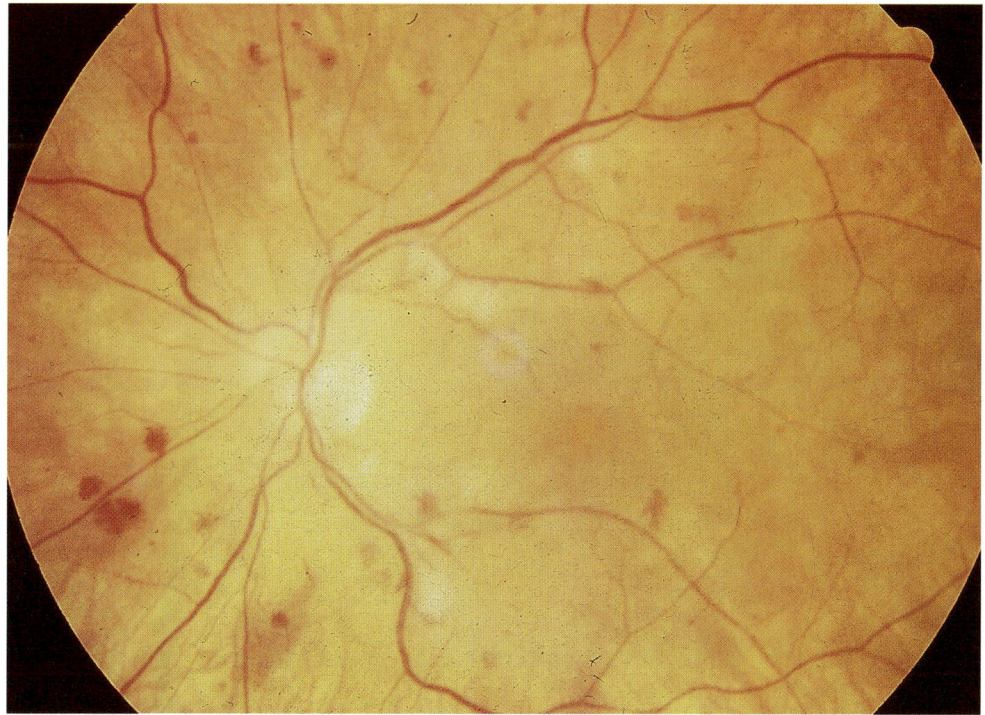

Figure 39 Funduscopy showing background retinopathy in a patient with diabetes mellitus. There are dot-and-blot hemorrhages, but no evidence of new-vessel formation. Hypertension accelerates microvascular disease in diabetes, and obesity, insulin resistance and hypertension are often coexistent

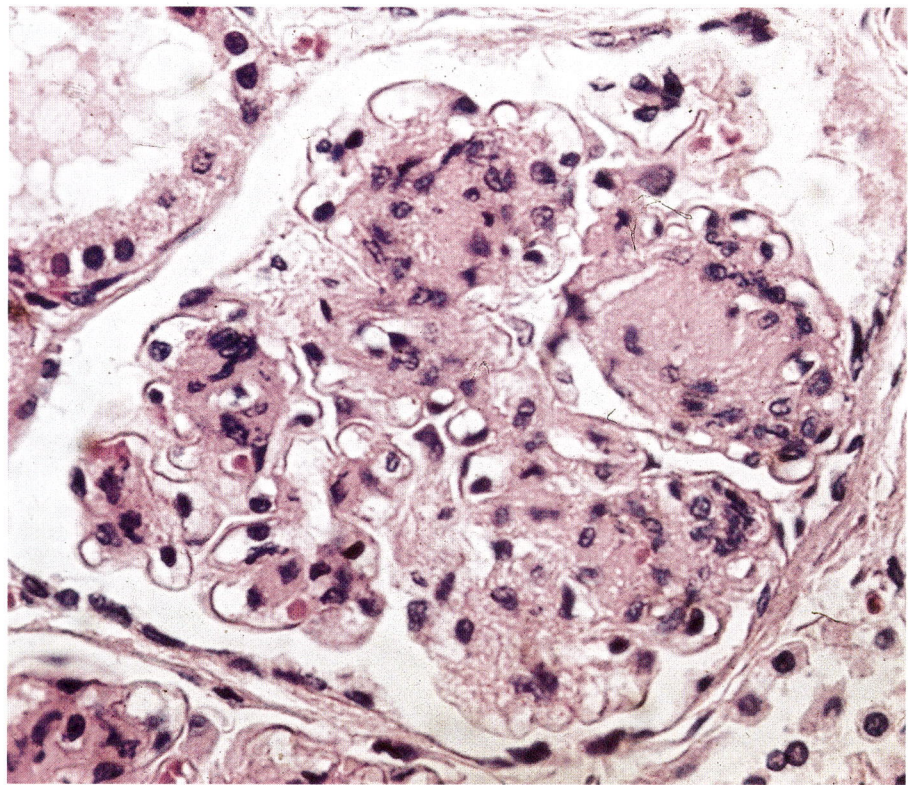

Figure 40 Histology of a renal glomerulus in a patient with long-standing diabetes mellitus shows several stages in the formation of Kimmelstiel–Wilson nodules in the mesangium of several lobules (H & E)

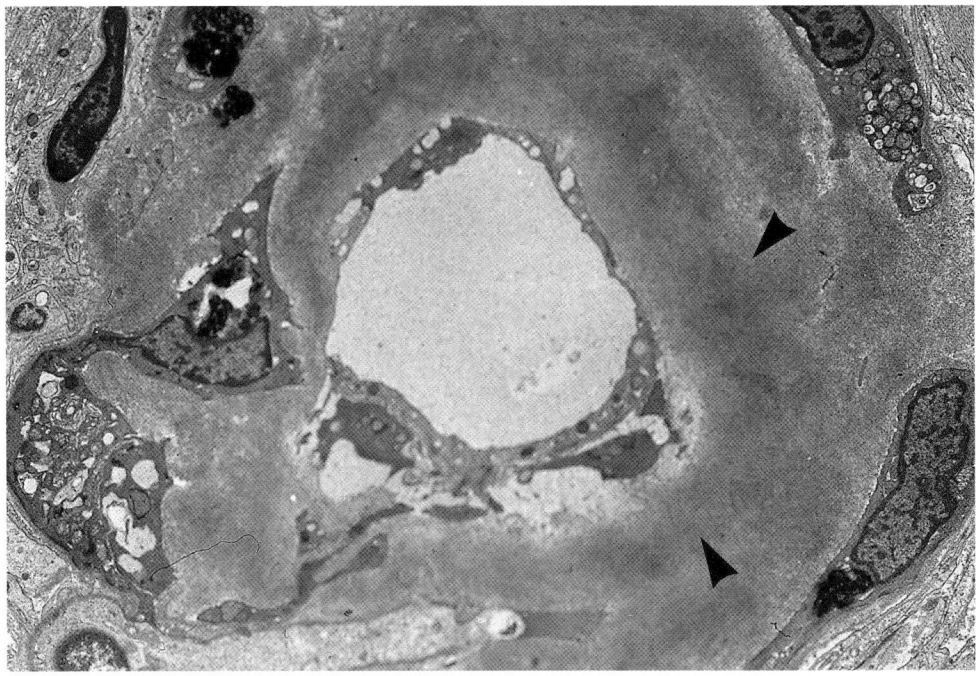

Figure 41 EM of an arteriole in diabetic microvascular disease shows replacement of medial smooth muscle cells by homogeneous deposits (arrowed) of material resembling basement membrane. These deposits are probably derived from both synthesis of excess basement membrane material and accumulation of proteins from plasma

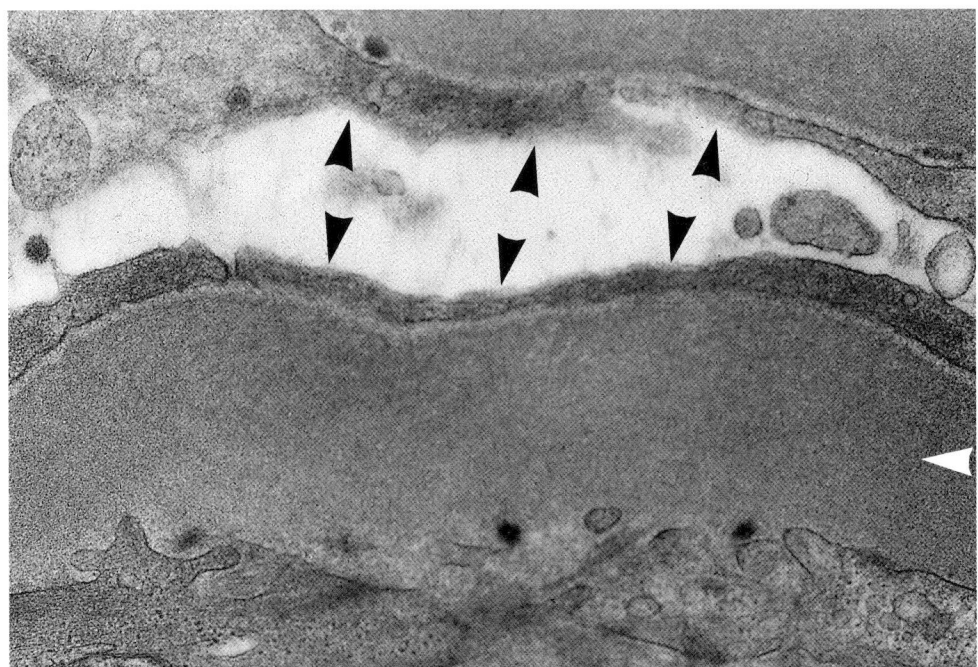

Figure 42 EM of a glomerular capillary wall in diabetes shows gross thickening of the basement membrane, seen as a homogeneous band (white arrow). There is also fusion (black arrows) of the foot processes of the podocyte

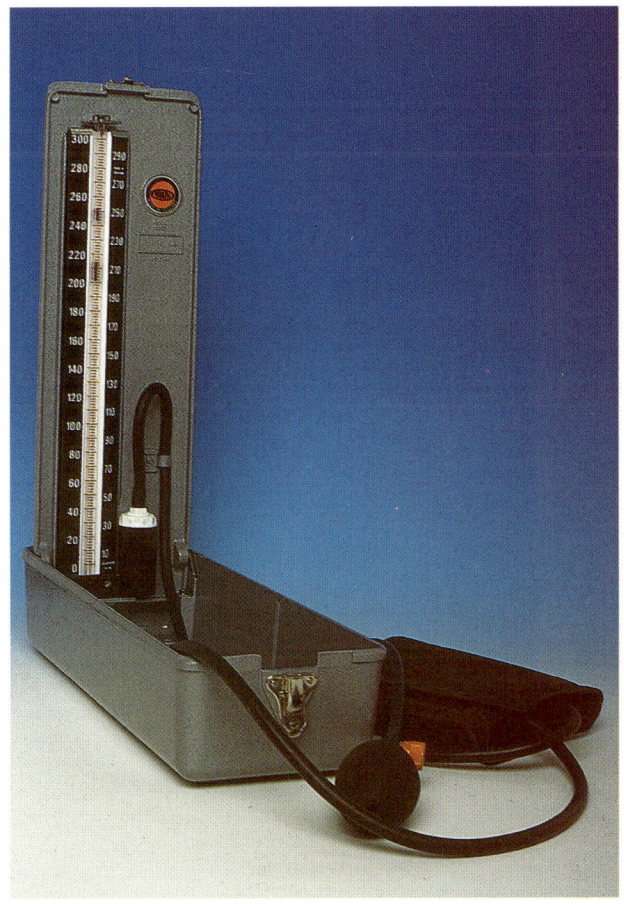

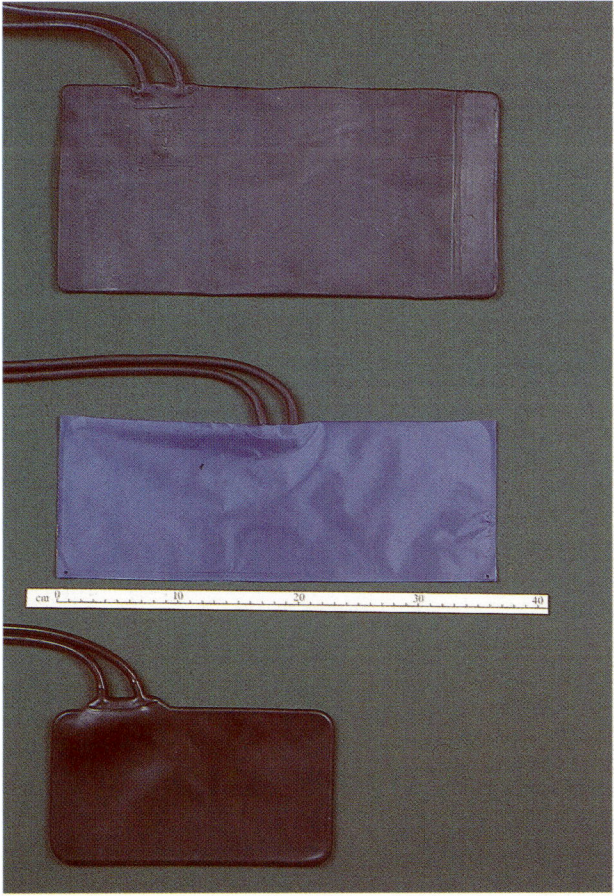

Figure 43 The mercury sphygmomanometer remains the standard instrument for measurement of blood pressure. Common remedial causes of inaccuracy are: the mercury meniscus does not start at zero; the inside of the glass tube is black; and the valve is not functioning properly. It should be possible to adjust the rate of descent of the mercury meniscus to 2 mm / s or less

Figure 44 Mercury sphygmomanometer bladders come in different sizes. The standard cuff for blood pressure measurement uses a bladder that is 35 cm in length (middle), which is longer than the traditional bladder (22 cm; lower). When using the 22-cm bladder, it is important to center the cuff accurately over the brachial artery. If the bladder is too short for an obese arm, then blood pressure will be overestimated

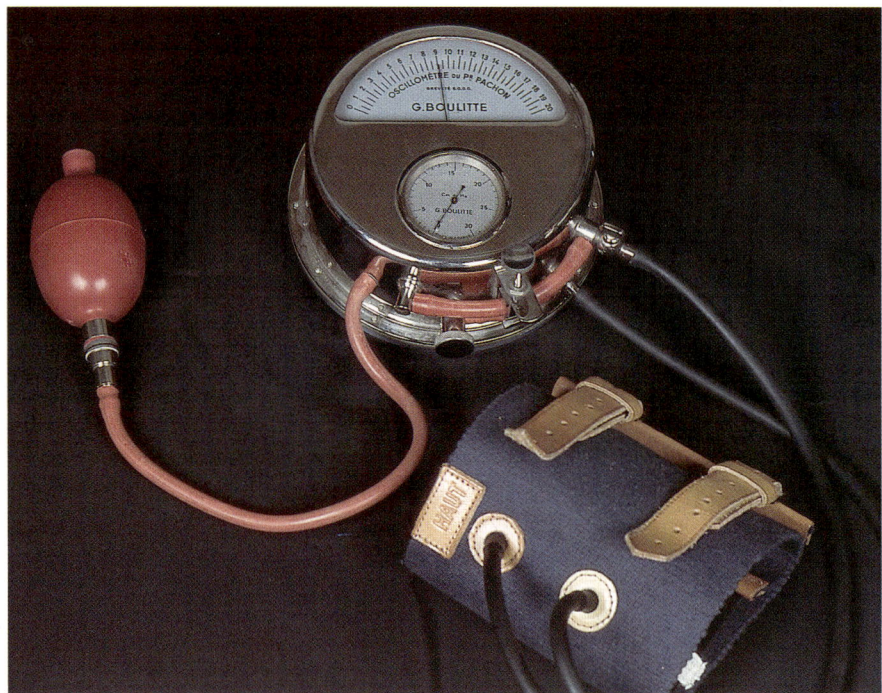

Figure 45 The Pachon oscillometer (first described in 1909) was a popular instrument for measuring blood pressure in the 1920s and 1930s. Oscillometry is the basis of some of the most widely used systems of non-invasive ambulatory blood pressure monitoring

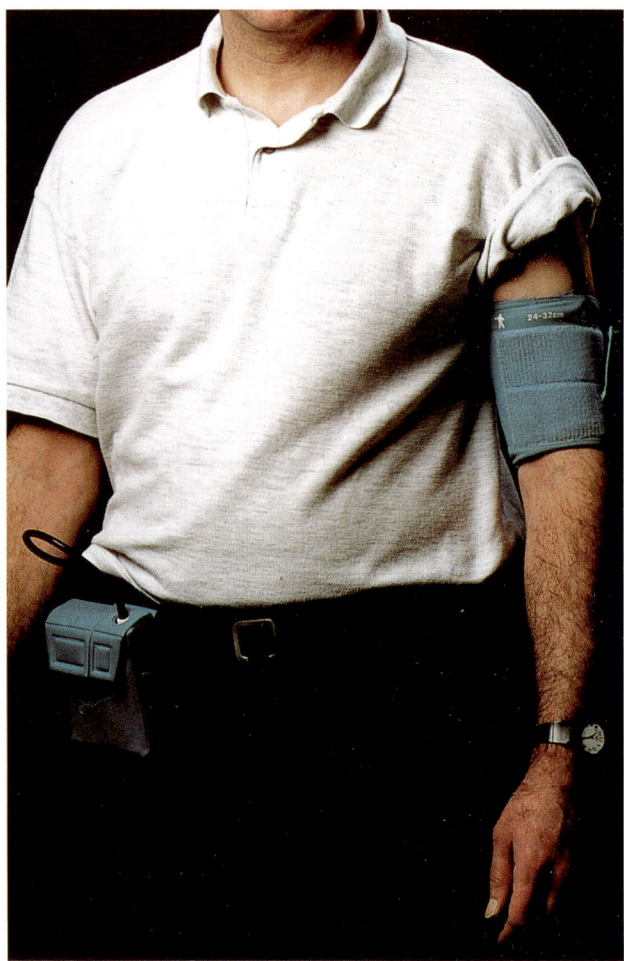

Figure 46 Contemporary equipment for the indirect measurement of ambulatory blood pressures

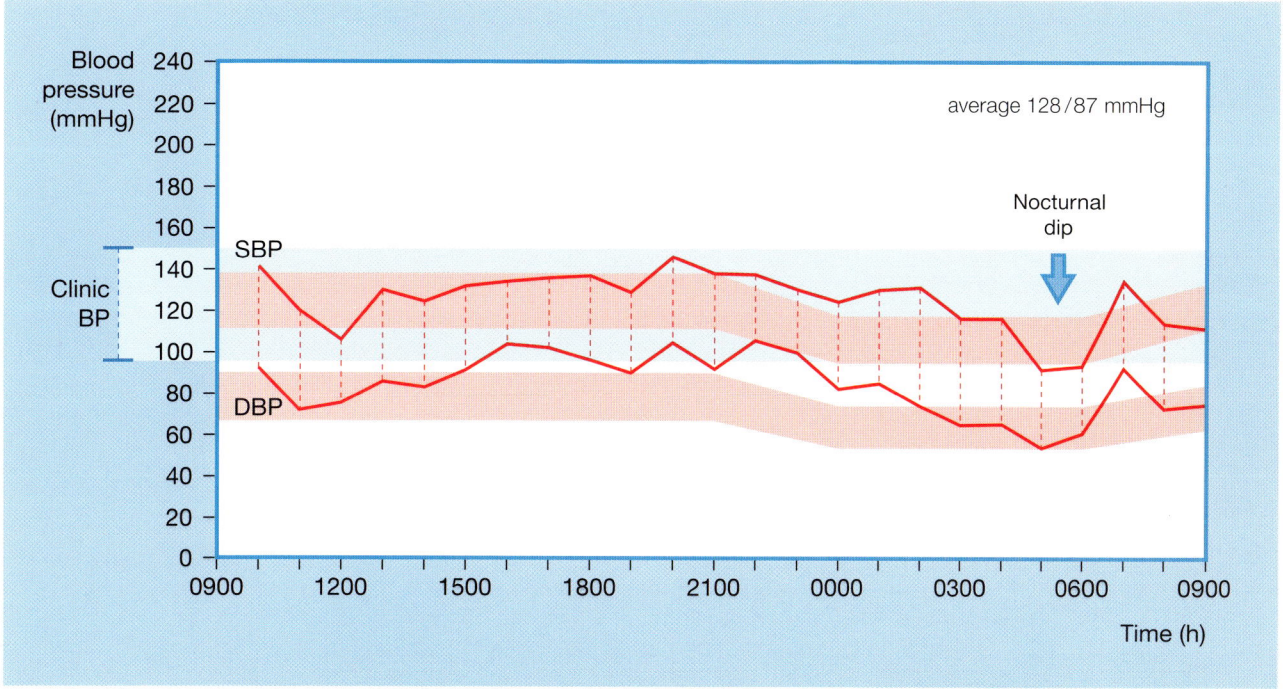

Figure 47 Pattern of 24-h ambulatory blood pressures in a patient with a sitting clinic pressure of 154/96 mmHg. Normal values are as determined by O'Brien *et al.* *J Hypertens* 1991;9:355–60. Diastolic blood pressures are probably mildly raised during the day, but there is a nocturnal dip

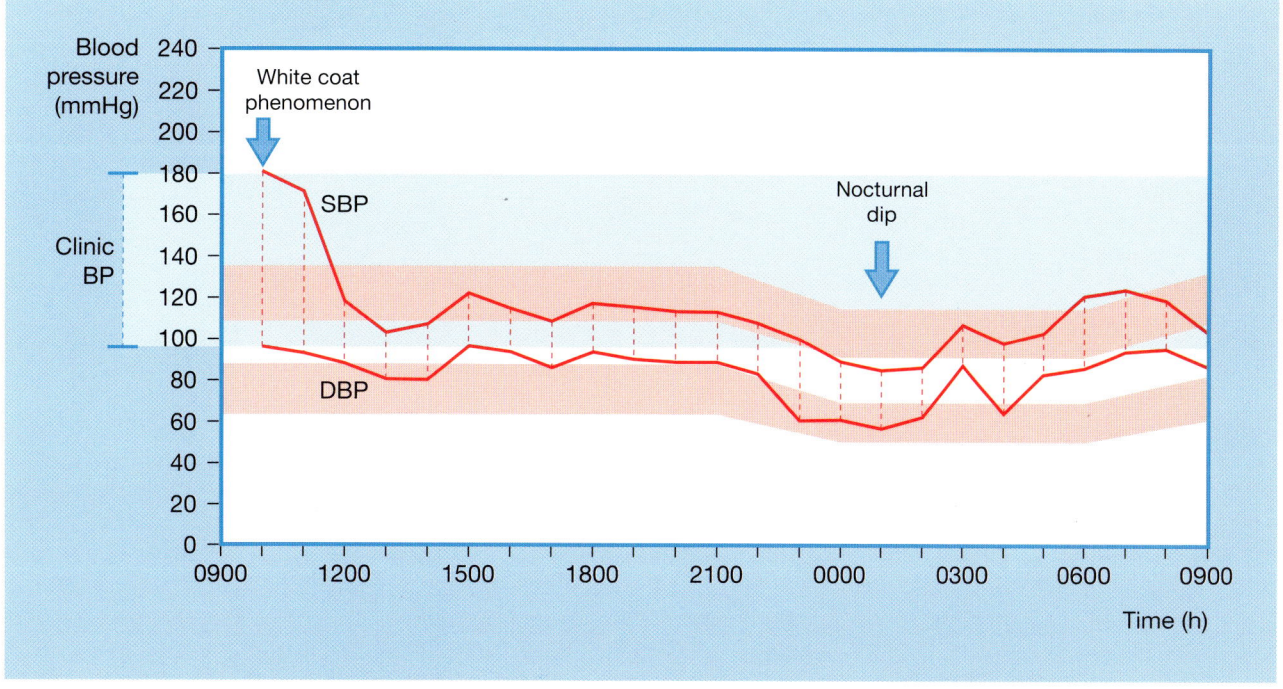

Figure 48 Pattern of 24-h ambulatory blood pressures in a patient with white-coat hypertension. Clinic blood pressure was 182/96 mmHg, but the mean 24-h pressure was only 109/81 mmHg

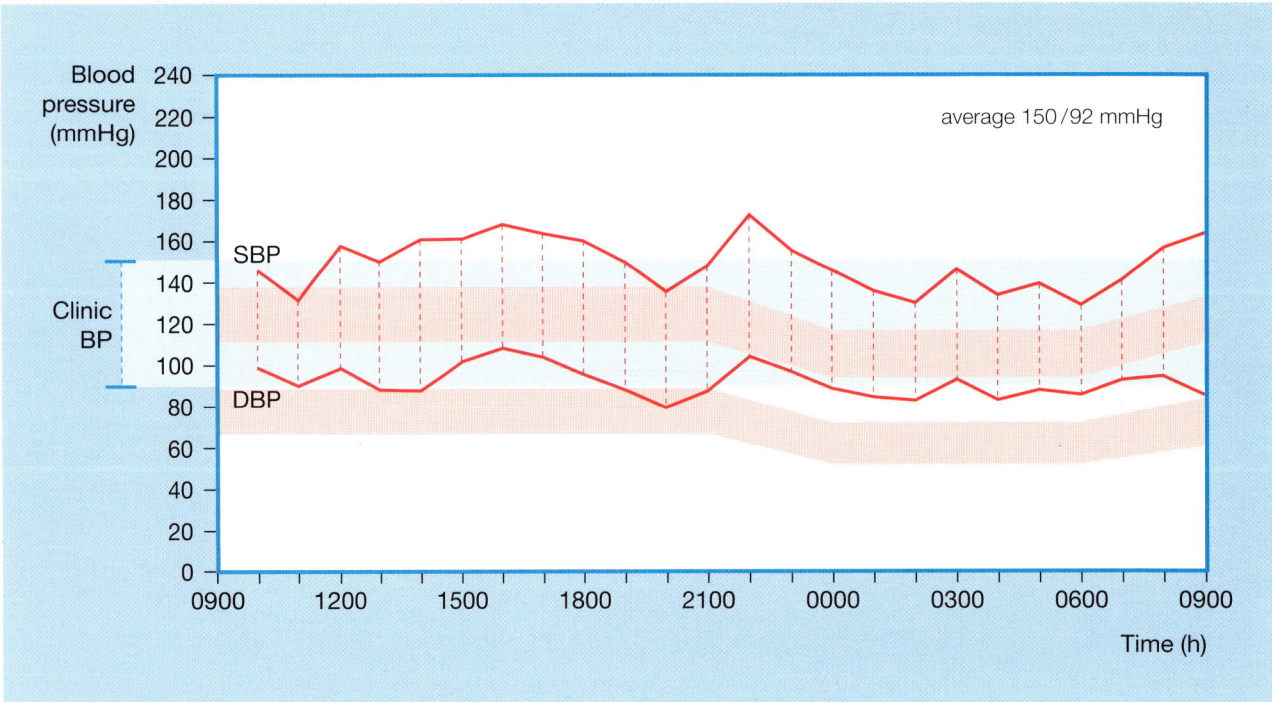

Figure 49 Pattern of 24-h ambulatory blood pressures confirms high values with a minor nocturnal dip. There is some evidence that lack of a nocturnal dip signifies a higher risk

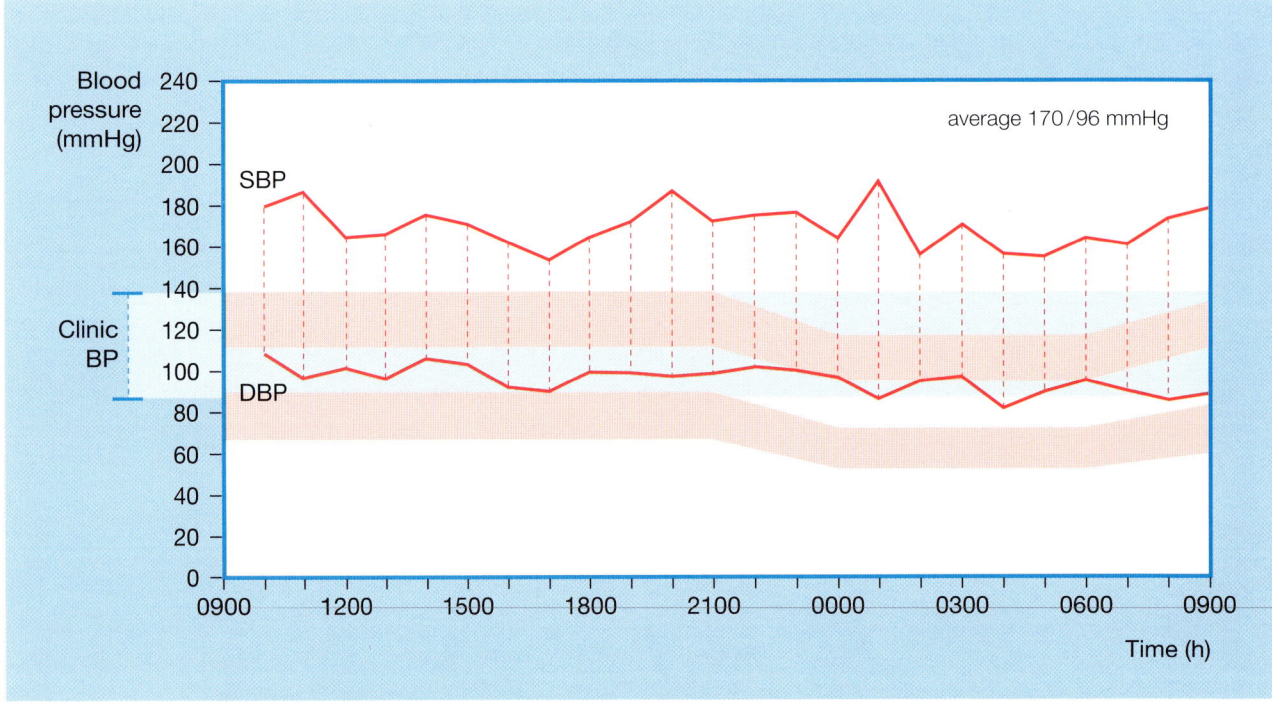

Figure 50 These 24-h ambulatory blood pressures are higher than the clinic pressure, which was 148/86 mmHg. There is no nocturnal dip. Ambulatory pressures are better predictors of LVH than are clinic measurements

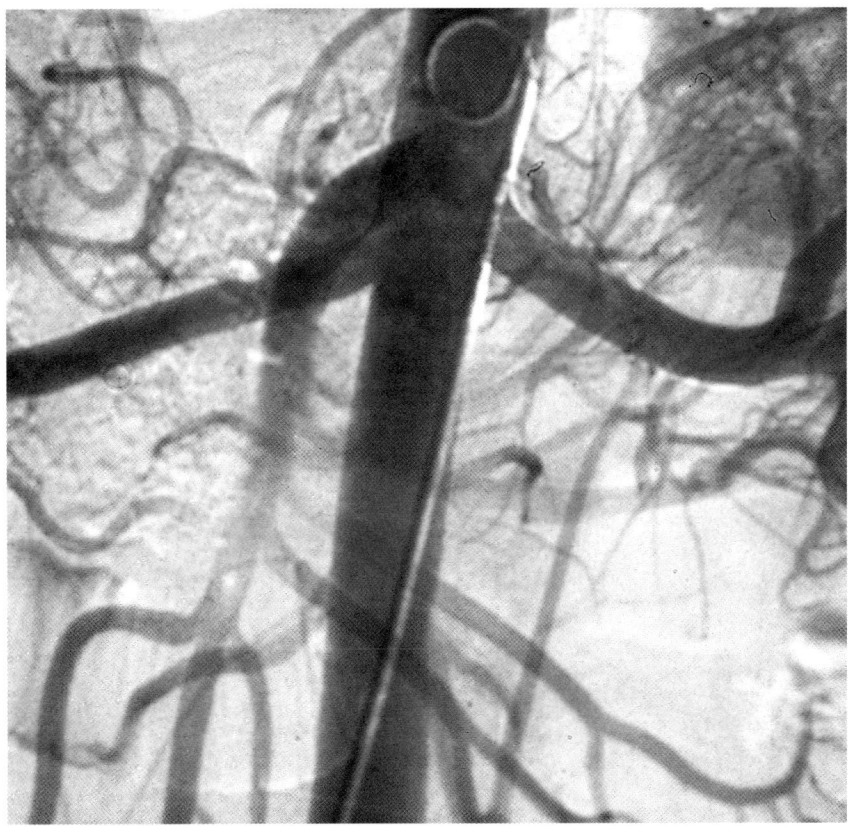

Figure 51 Digital subtraction angiogram after aortic flush injection showing normal renal arteries

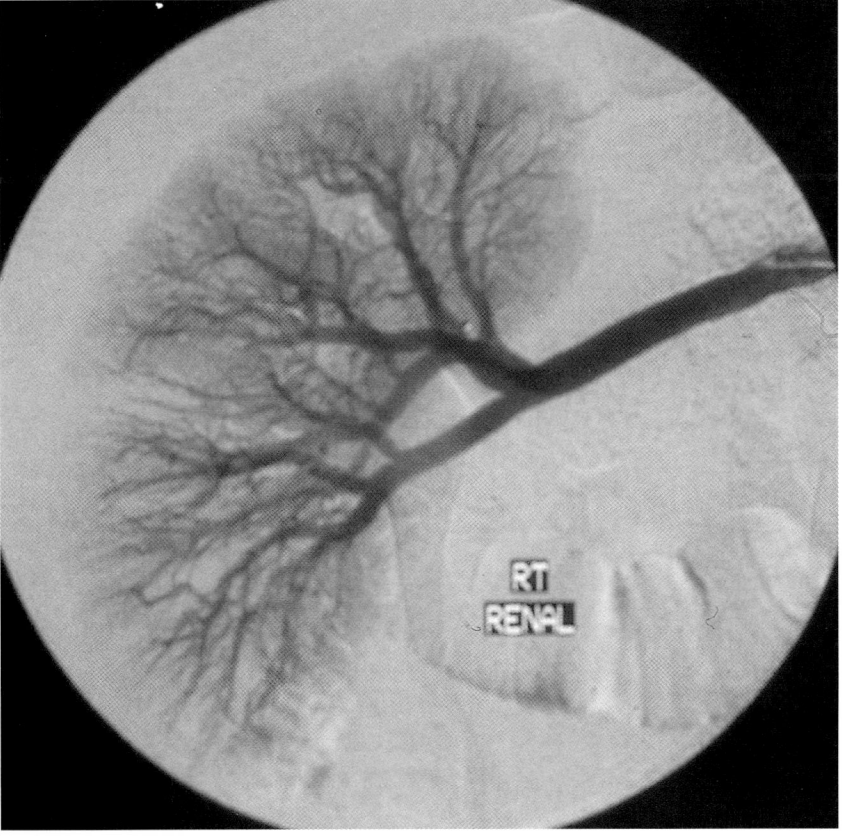

Figure 52 Modern digital subtraction angiogram is able to show intrarenal arteries clearly, as seen in this normal examination

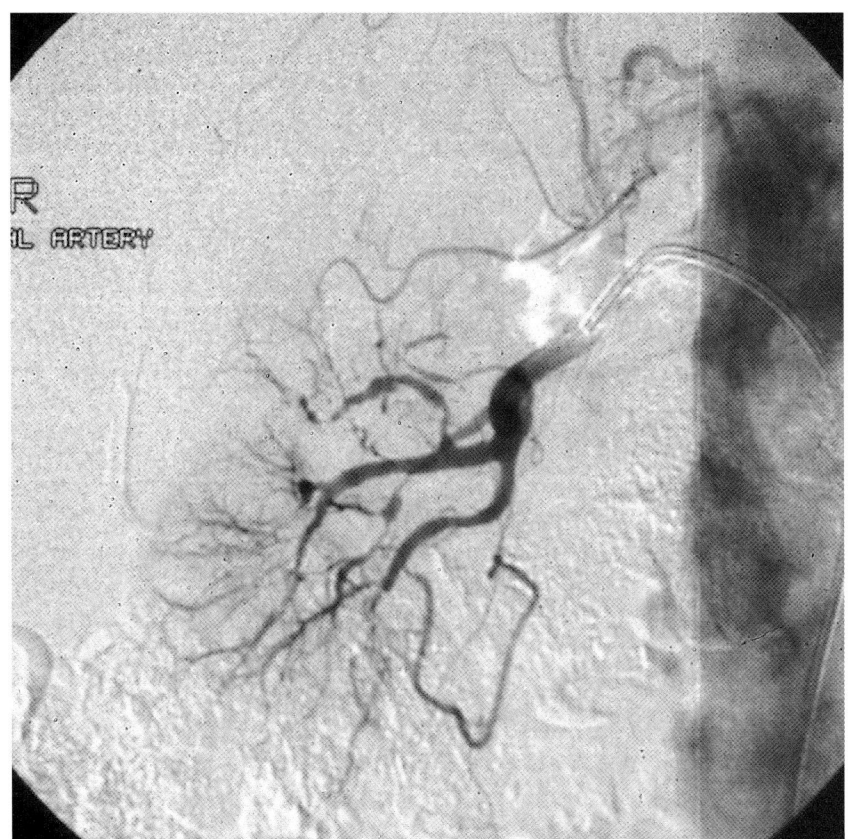

Figure 53 Digital subtraction arteriogram of a kidney from a patient with renal impairment caused by longstanding hypertension. The architecture of the intrarenal arteries is highly abnormal, and there is rarefaction, pruning and variation in arterial caliber

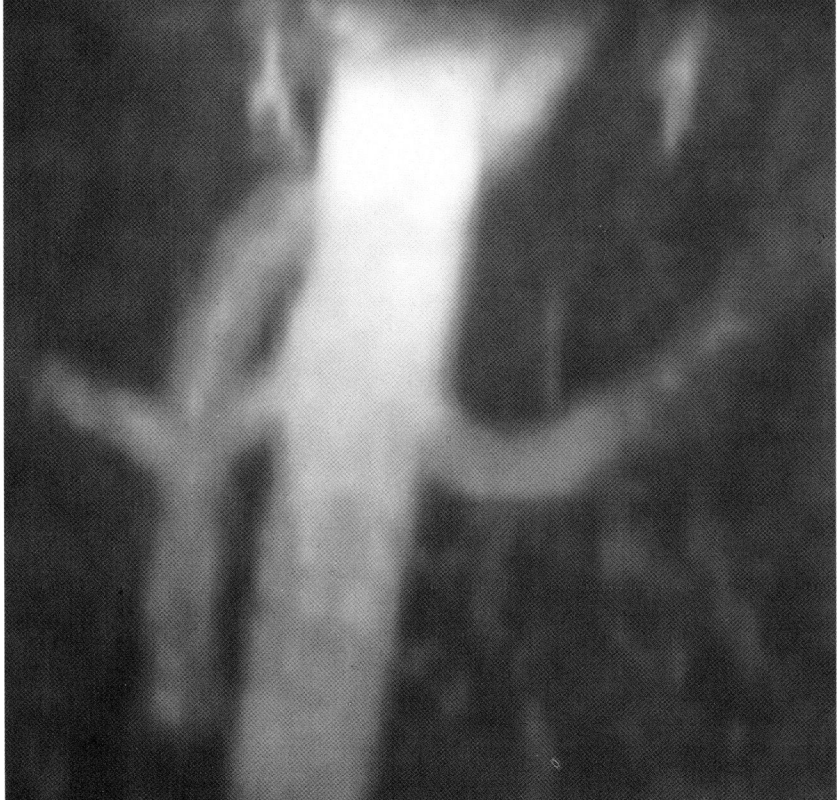

Figure 54 MRI showing abdominal aorta and normal renal arteries. MRI is entirely non-invasive, but contrast examinations still provide better definition

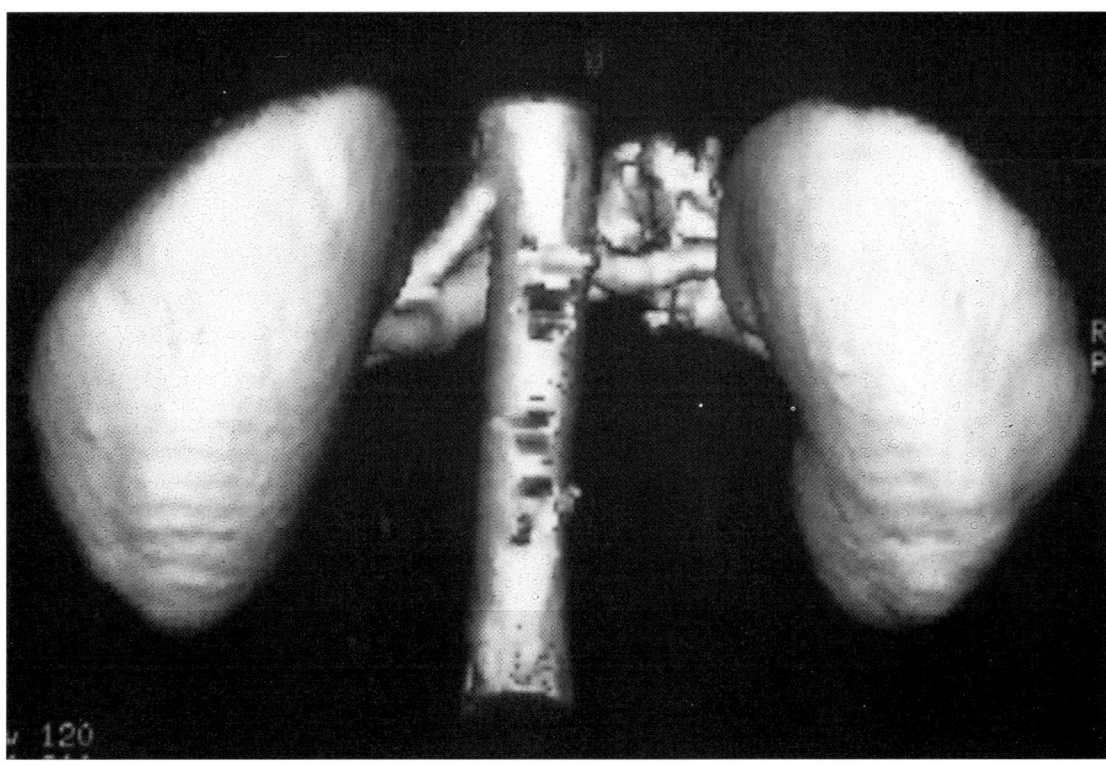

Figure 55 Surface reconstruction of a spiral CT angiogram showing a normal aorta and renal vasculature in a three-dimensional (3-D) image

right renal artery
stenosis

left renal artery
stenosis

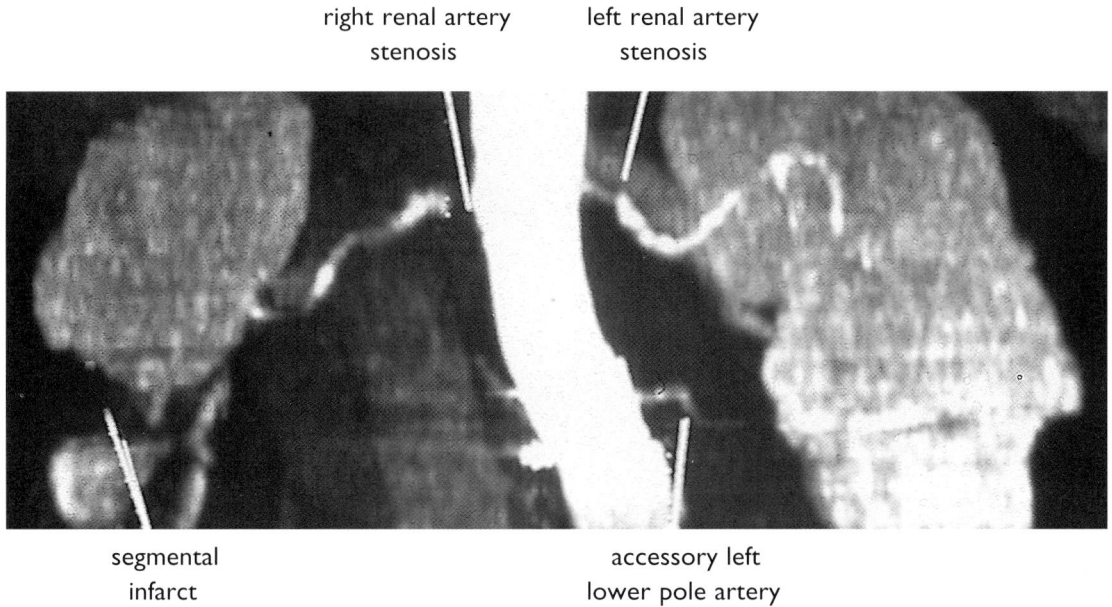

segmental
infarct

accessory left
lower pole artery

Figure 56 Maximum-intensity projection of a spiral CT angiogram showing bilateral renal artery stenosis and infarction of the lower pole of the right kidney

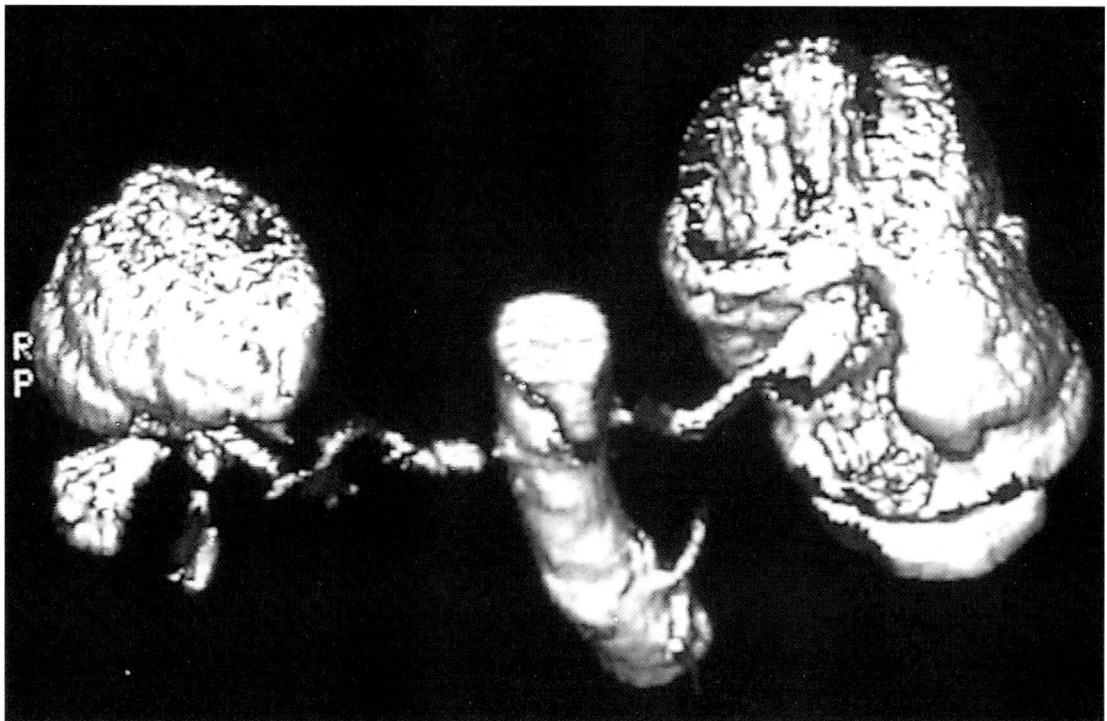

Figure 57 Surface reconstruction of a spiral CT angiogram (same scan as in Figure 56) produces a 3-D image of the aorta and renal vasculature. This modality is less effective than 2-D maximum-intensity projection in the diagnosis of renal artery stenosis

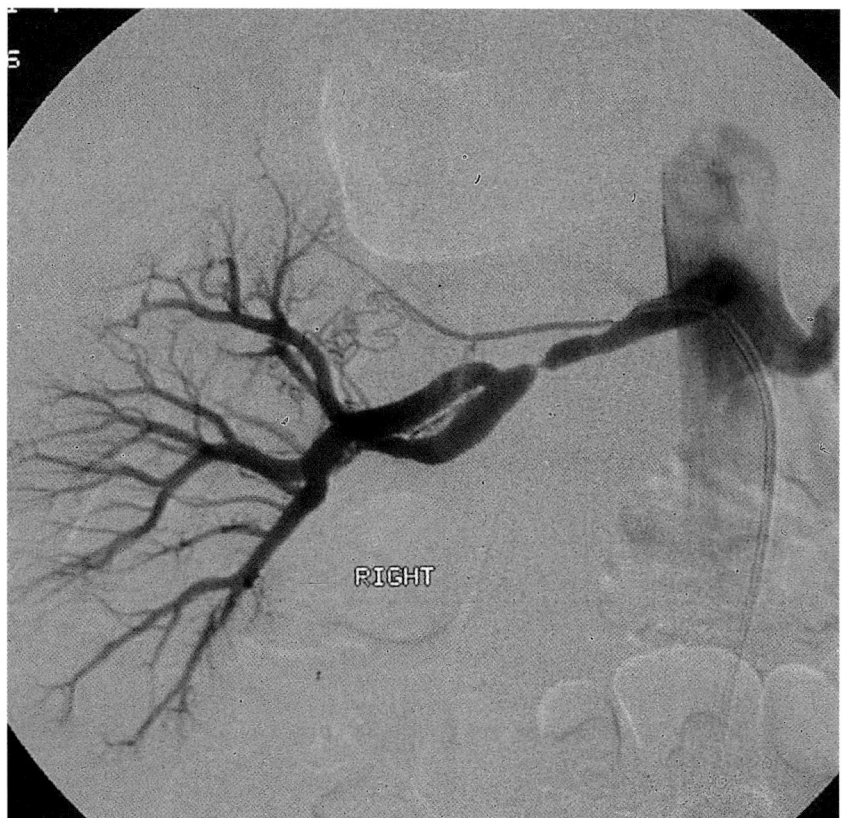

Figure 58 Digital subtraction angiogram showing a tight renal artery stenosis due to localized fibromuscular dysplasia in a 27-year-old nurse who had hypertension. Longer stenotic segments often present with a 'string-of-beads' appearance

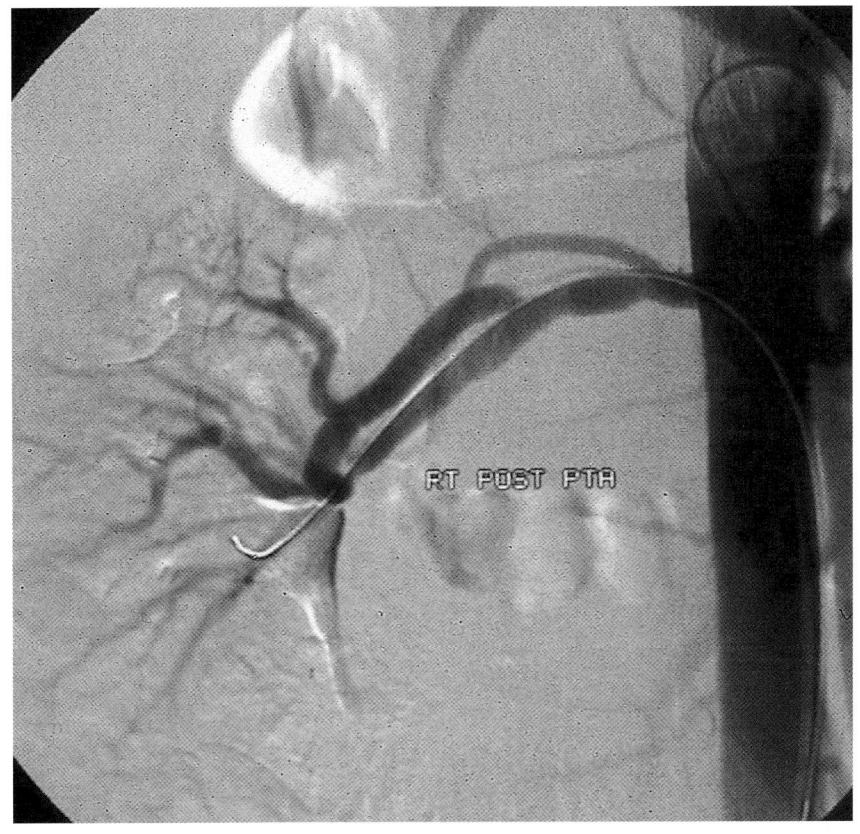

Figure 59 Digital subtraction angiogram of the same artery as in Figure 58 shown after successful percutaneous balloon angioplasty

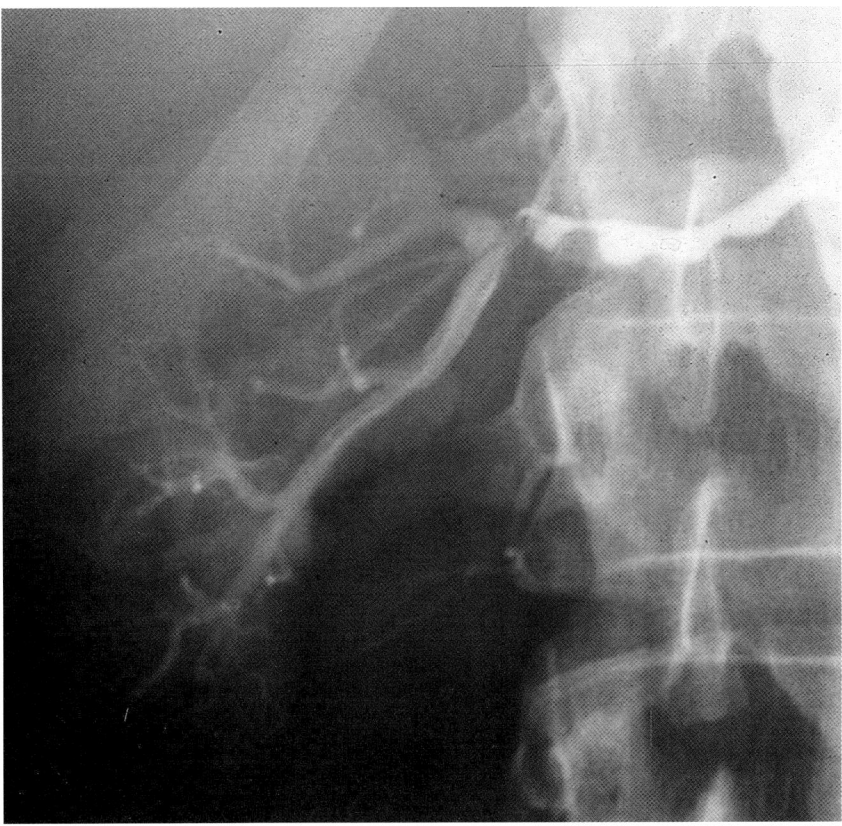

Figure 60 Angiogram of a right renal artery showing dissection and thrombosis in a segment with fibromuscular dysplasia. The patient was a young woman who had presented with loin pain and hypertension

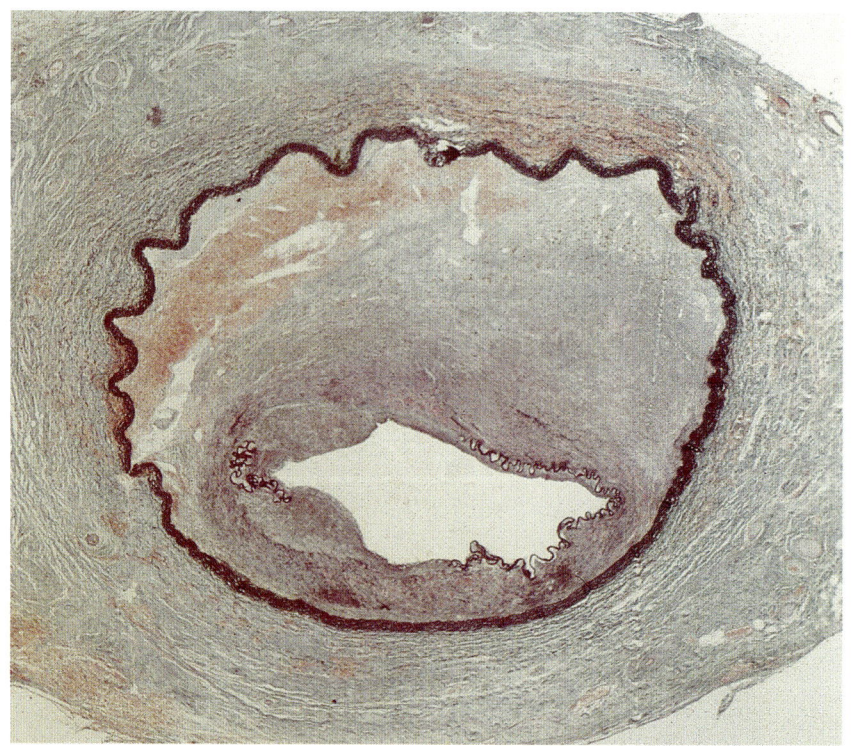

Figure 61 Histology showing a transverse section of a renal artery stained for elastic fibers (black). This appearance is typical of perimedial fibromuscular dysplasia. The internal elastic lamina (black) is fragmented, and some residual media is enclosed within the thicker external elastic lamina. A hematoma (stained reddish-brown) caused by arterial dissection lies below and to the left (elastica Martius scarlet–blue)

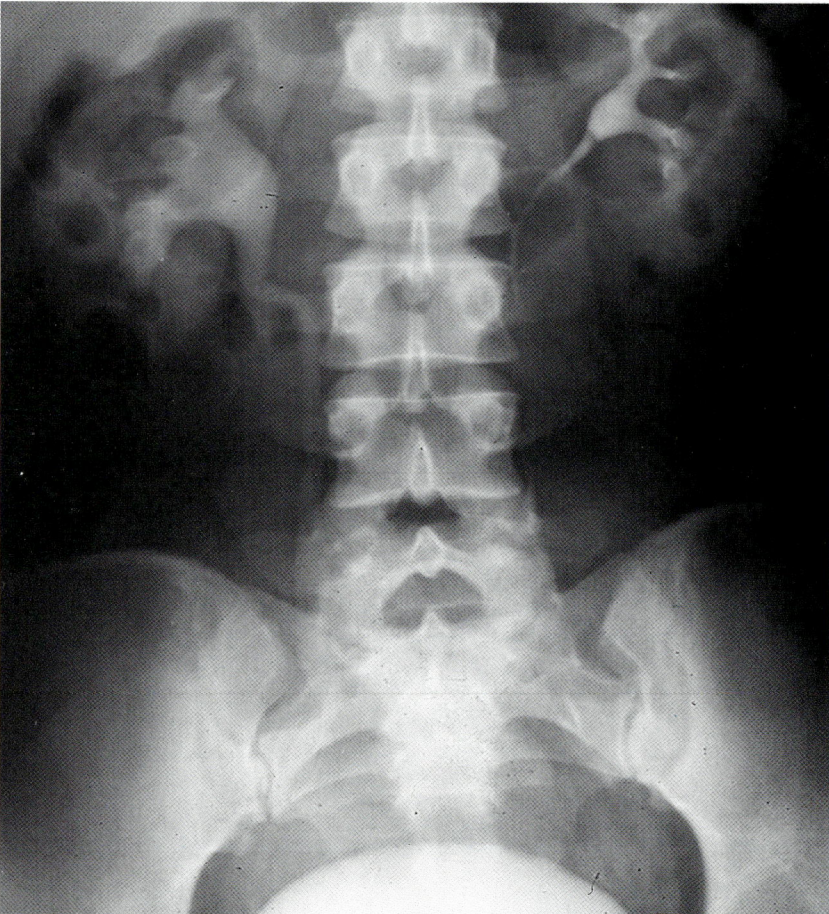

Figure 62 Intravenous urogram in a patient with left renal artery stenosis. There is an increased density of contrast in the collecting system of the affected kidney, which was slow to wash out after an oral water load. Urography has been superseded as a method of screening for renovascular hypertension

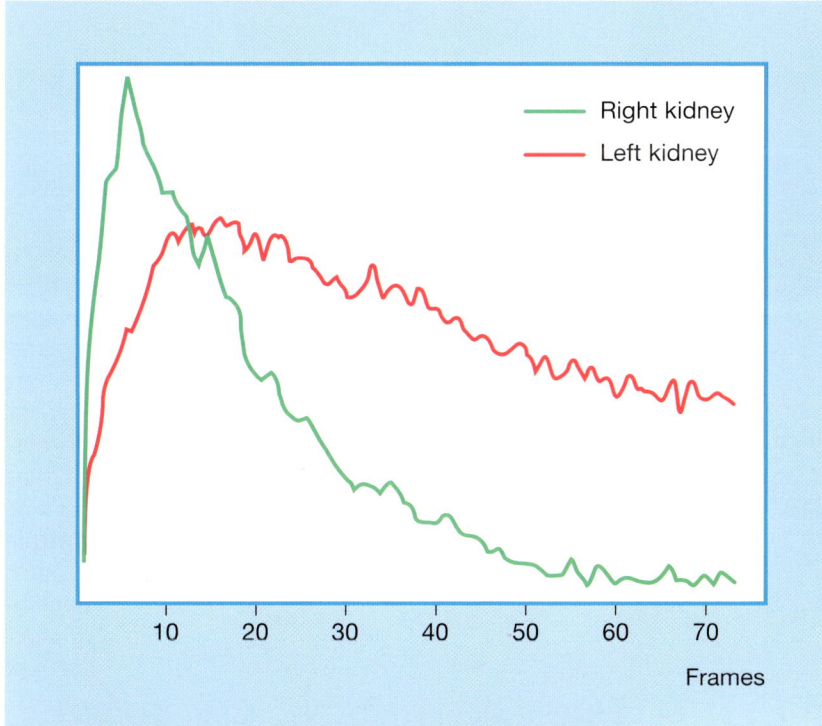

Figure 63 Graph showing the typical curves derived by captopril renography of a patient with left renal artery stenosis. The $t_{1/2}$ and t_{max} are characteristically prolonged. The method is useful for detecting unilateral functional renal artery stenosis

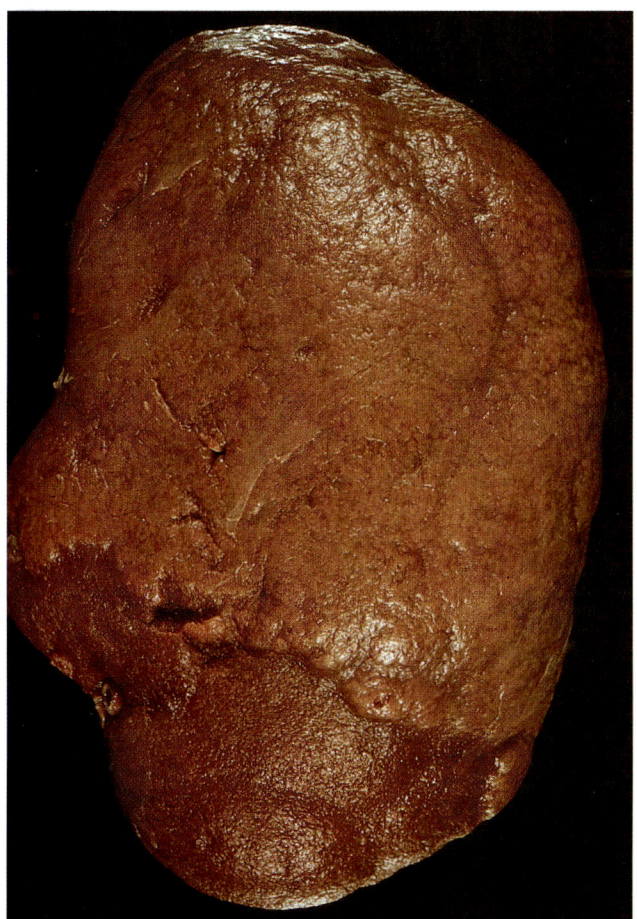

Figure 64 Kidney with stenosis of the artery supplying the lower pole, which is shrunken and contracted. Typically, the affected part of the kidney is darker red and more granular than the adjacent normal kidney tissue

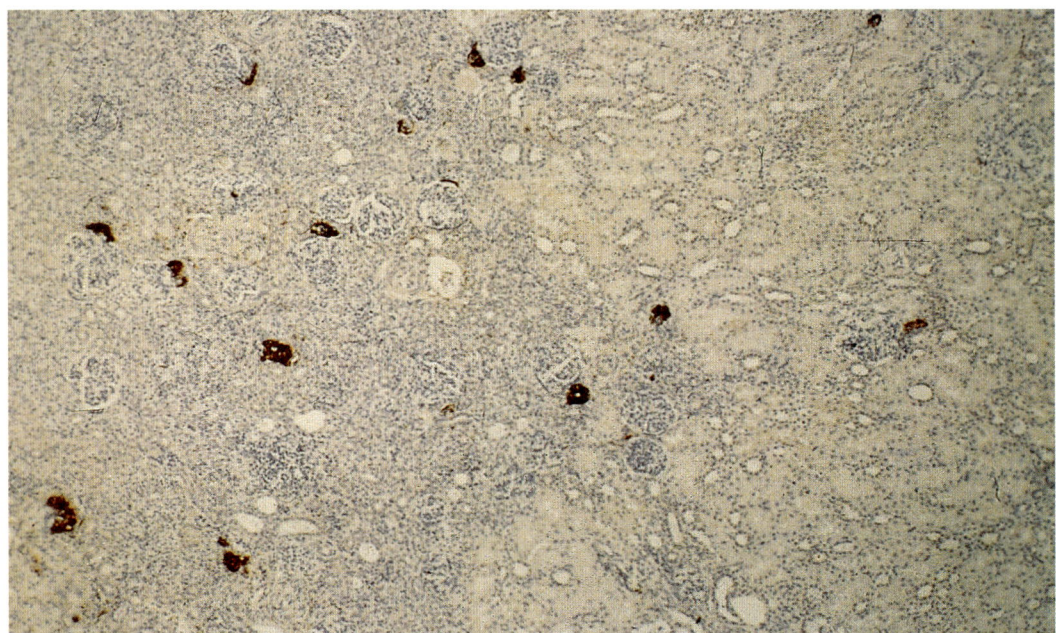

Figure 65 Histology of a kidney showing the junction of ischemic (to the left) and normal (to the right) renal cortex. There is an abundance of brown-staining immuno-stainable renin in hyperplastic juxtaglomerular apparatuses in the ischemic areas, and diminished renin in the normal tissue as a result of suppression of renin synthesis (immunoperoxidase technique)

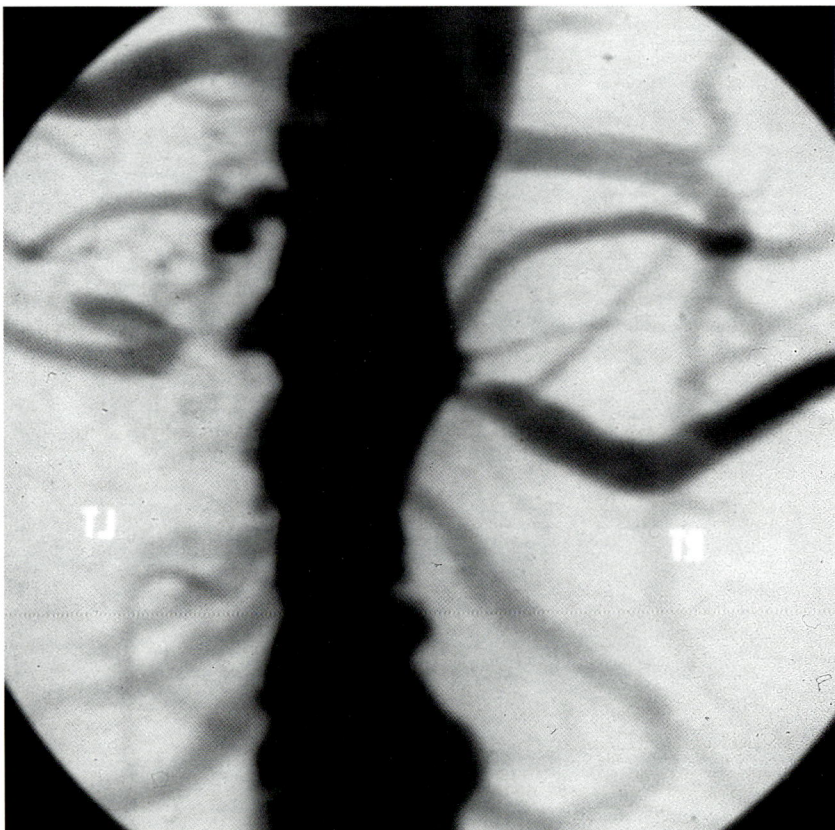

Figure 66 Digital subtraction angiogram of the aorta and renal vasculature showing a left renal artery that has been reduced to a stump due to arterial occlusion; the right renal artery has a stenosis at its origin. Patients with bilateral renal artery disease are liable to renal failure after treatment with either angiotensin-converting enzyme inhibitors or angiotensin-receptor antagonists

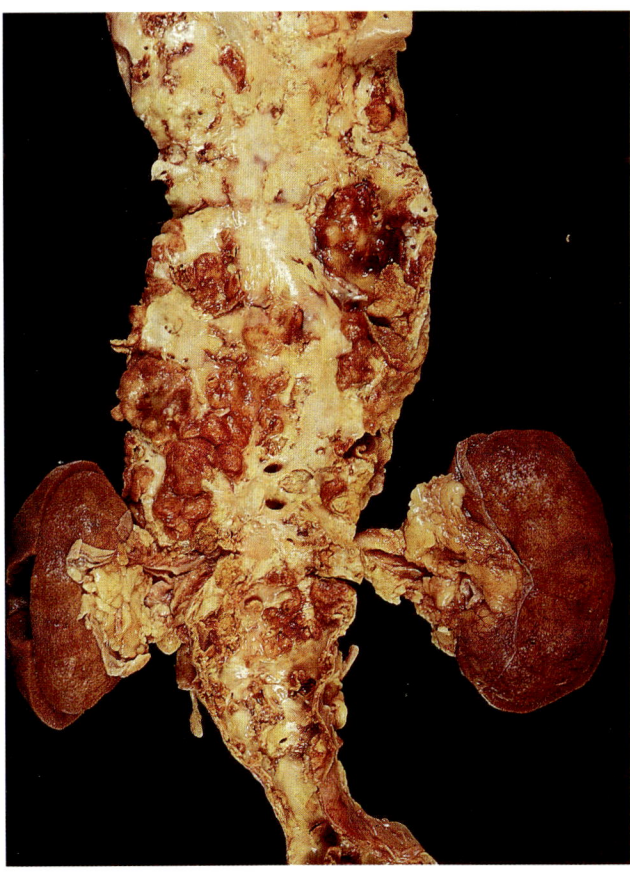

Figure 67 Postmortem abdominal aorta and kidneys showing ulcerating aortic atheroma, which may cause cholesterol embolism in life. Clinical manifestations of cholesterol embolism include renal impairment, livido reticularis and ischemic areas in the toes

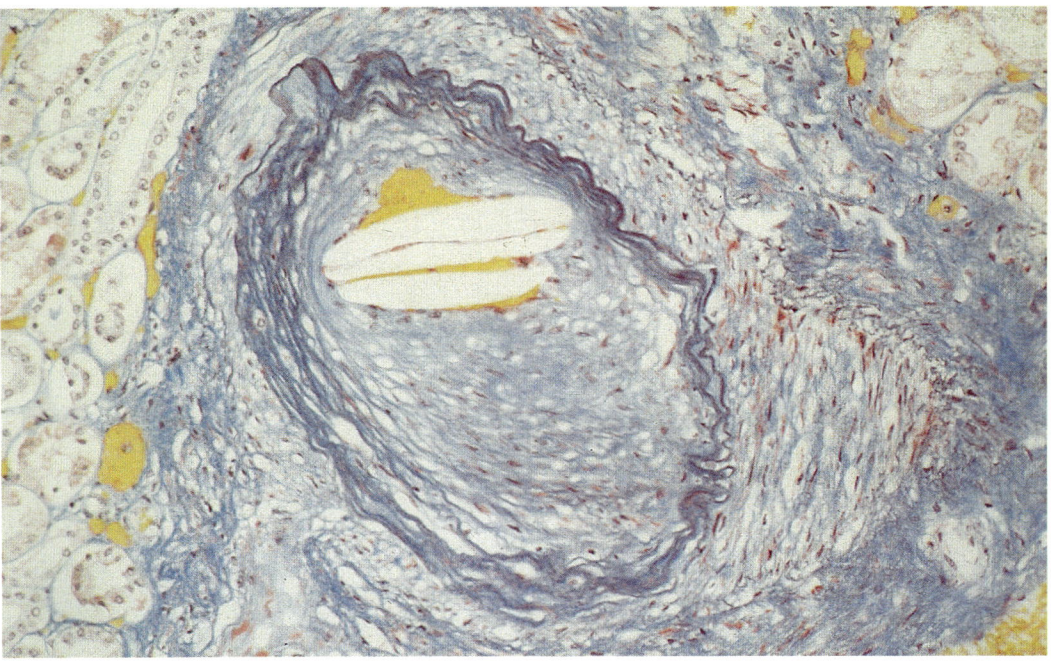

Figure 68 Histology showing transverse section of a renal artery with athero-embolism. The clefts in the lumen were caused by dissolution of cholesterol crystals during preparation of the tissue for microscopy (H & E)

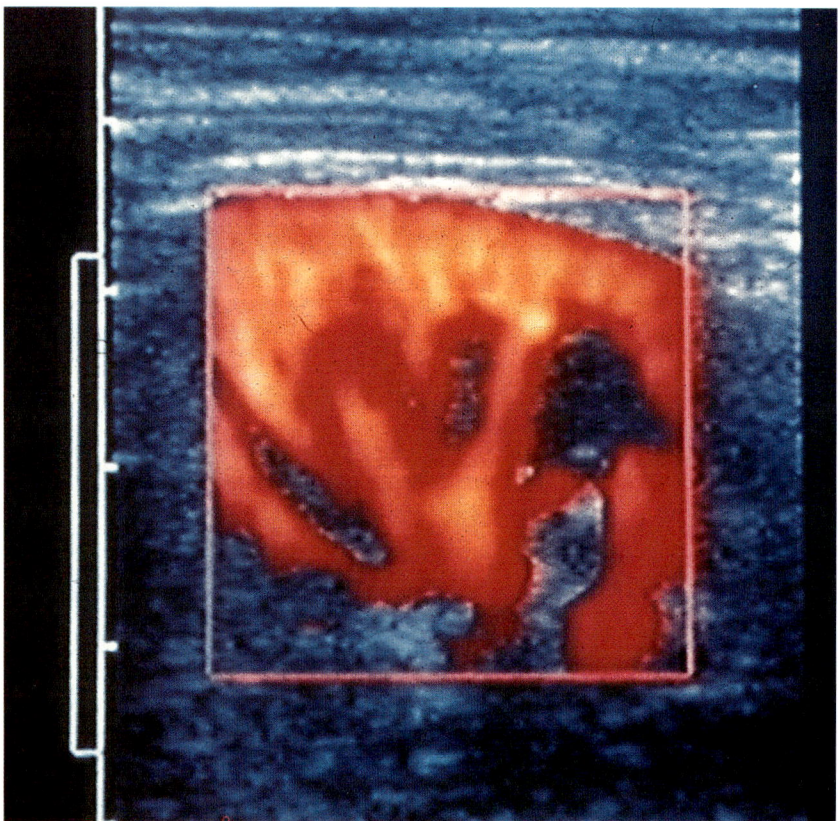

Figure 69 Power Doppler shows the interlobar arteries of the kidney, which show reduced pulsatility distal to renal artery stenosis

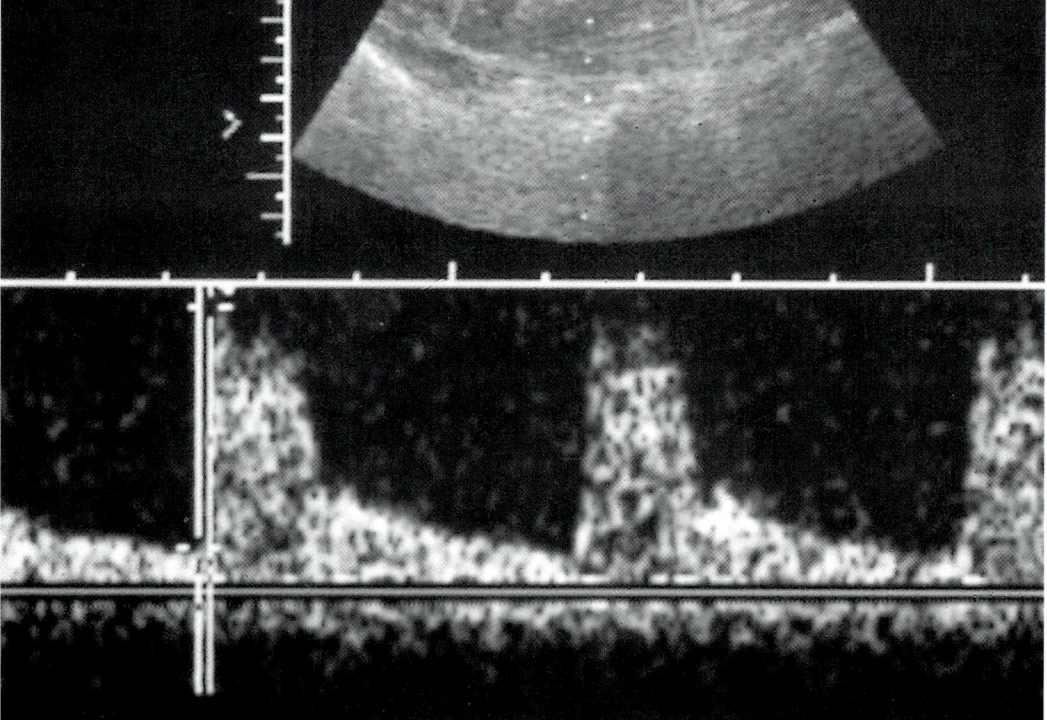

Figure 70 Doppler flow signature (below) from a normal interlobar artery shows a sharp upstroke with a well-defined peak and biphasic descent

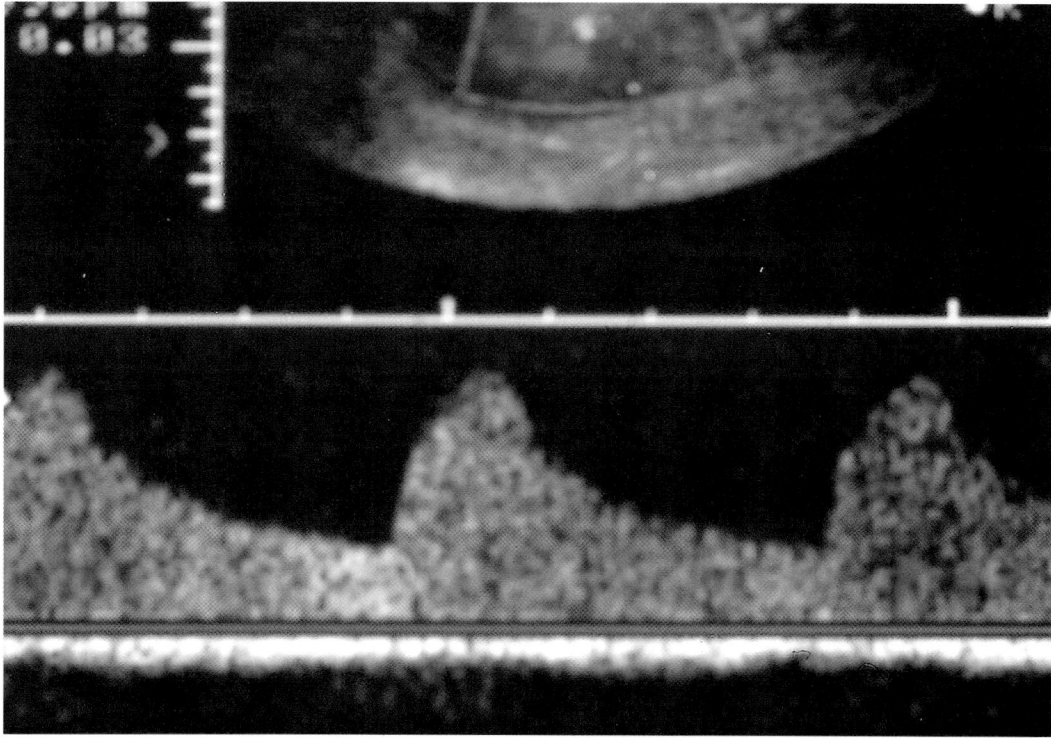

Figure 71 Doppler flow signature (below) from an interlobar artery distal to a renal artery stenosis is abnormal. The rounded contour is an expression of reduced pulsatility. This non-invasive technique may be useful in the diagnosis and detection of restenosis after angioplasty

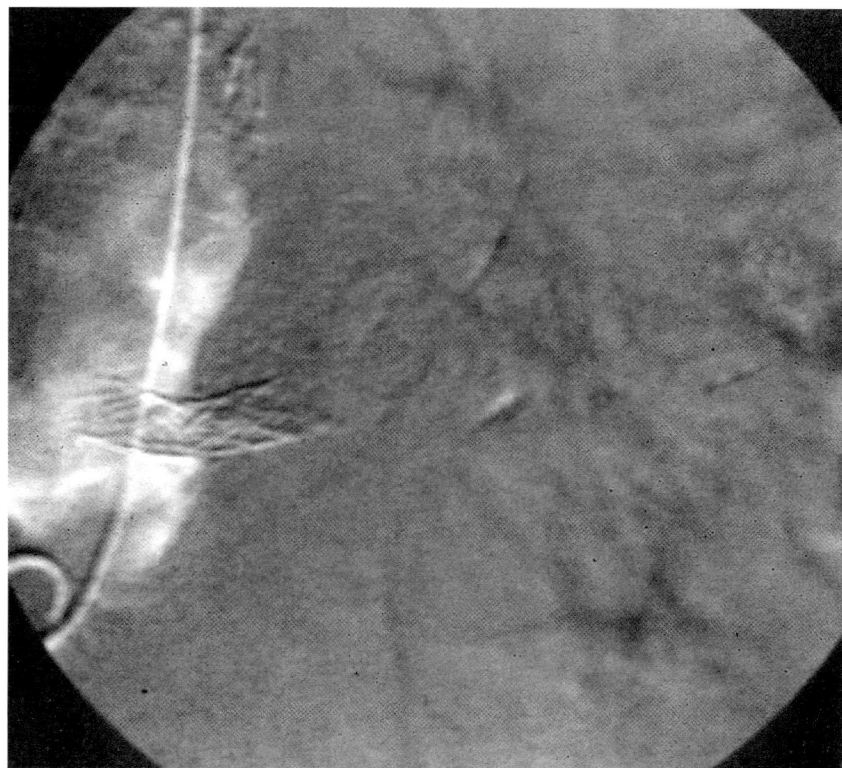

Figure 72 Digital subtraction angiogram showing an endovascular stent at the origin of the renal artery. Stents are of particular value in the treatment of patients with ostial renal artery stenosis

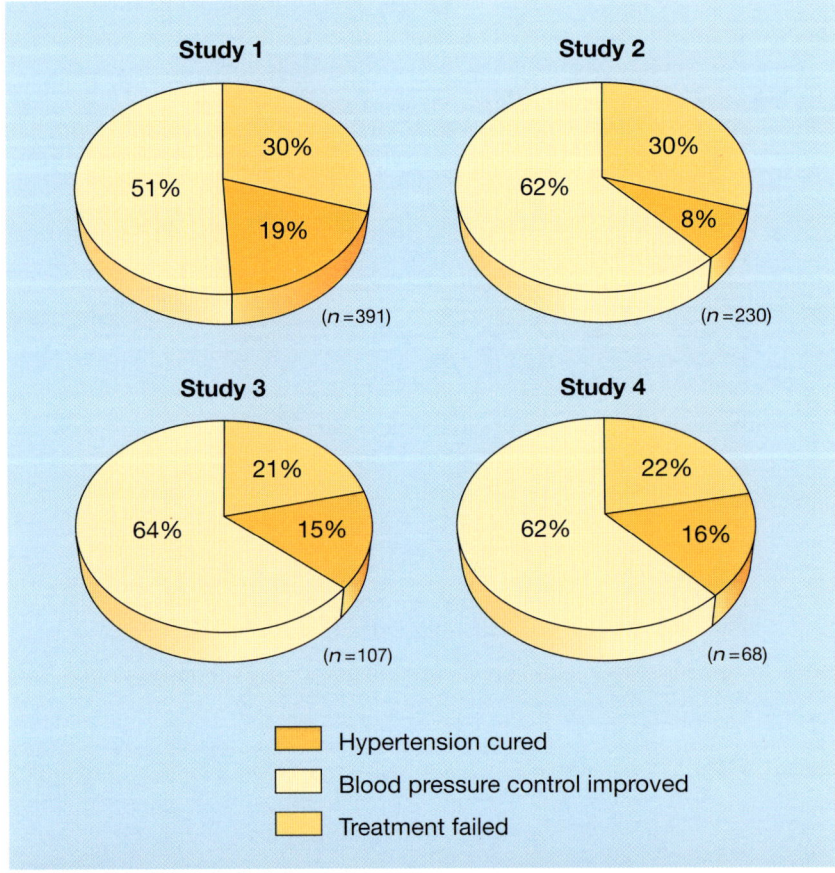

Study 1

30%

19%

51%

(*n*=391)

Study 2

30%

8%

62%

(*n*=230)

Study 3

21%

15%

64%

(*n*=107)

Study 4

22%

16%

62%

(*n*=68)

- ▣ Hypertension cured
- ▣ Blood pressure control improved
- ▣ Treatment failed

Figure 73 Graphs showing the results of studies (Study 1: Ramsey et al., *Br Med J* 1990;300:569–72; Study 2: Bonelli et al., *Mayo Clin Proc* 1995;70:1041–52; Study 3: Jensen et al., *Kidney Int* 1995;48: 1936–45; Study 4: Blum et al., *N Engl J Med* 1996;336:459–65) using angioplasty (or stents, as in Study 4) in the treatment of hypertension associated with atherosclerotic renal artery stenosis. Cure of hypertension in atherosclerotic renal artery stenosis is seldom achieved by angioplasty, although renal function may be improved or stabilized. The treatment of cases with fibromuscular dysplasia gives much better results

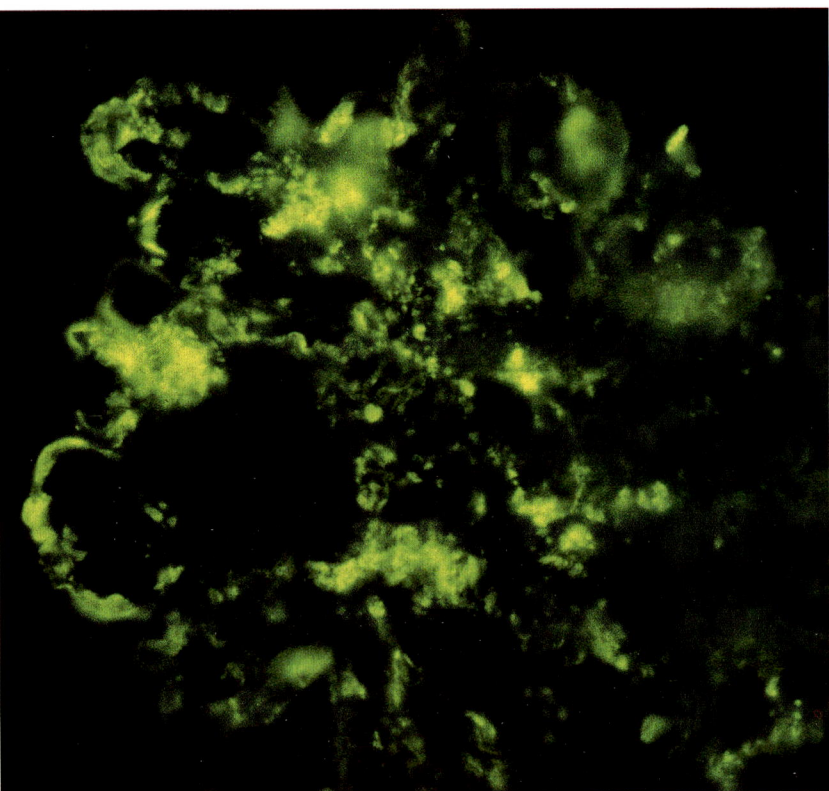

Figure 74 Immunofluorescence of a renal glomerulus showing granular deposits of IgA immune complex (yellow-green) mainly in the mesangium, typical of IgA nephropathy (Berger's disease). Patients with IgA nephropathy often present with hypertension, and are usually positive on urine stick tests for blood and protein

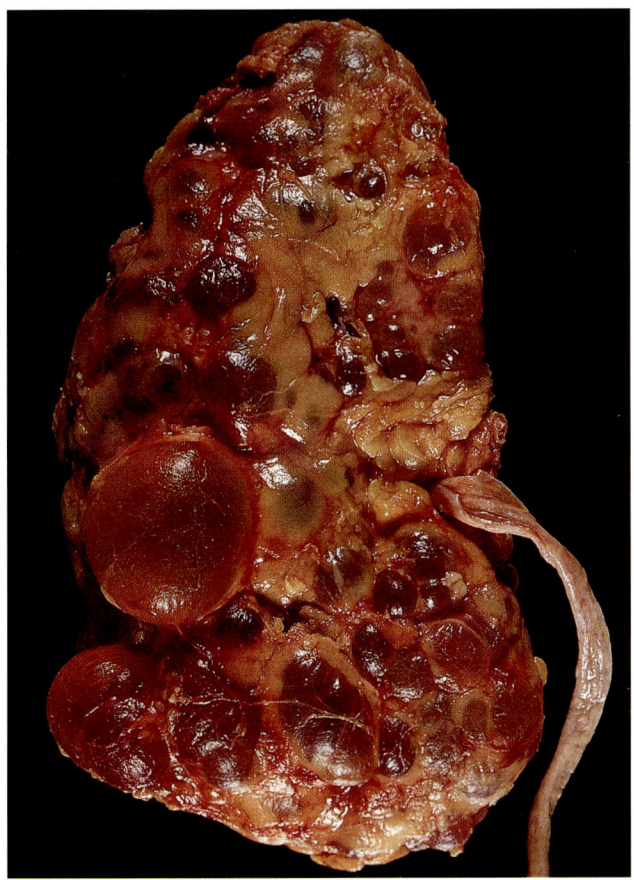

Figure 75 Kidney in autosomal-dominant (adult) polycystic kidney disease showing large cysts which have replaced normal kidney tissue

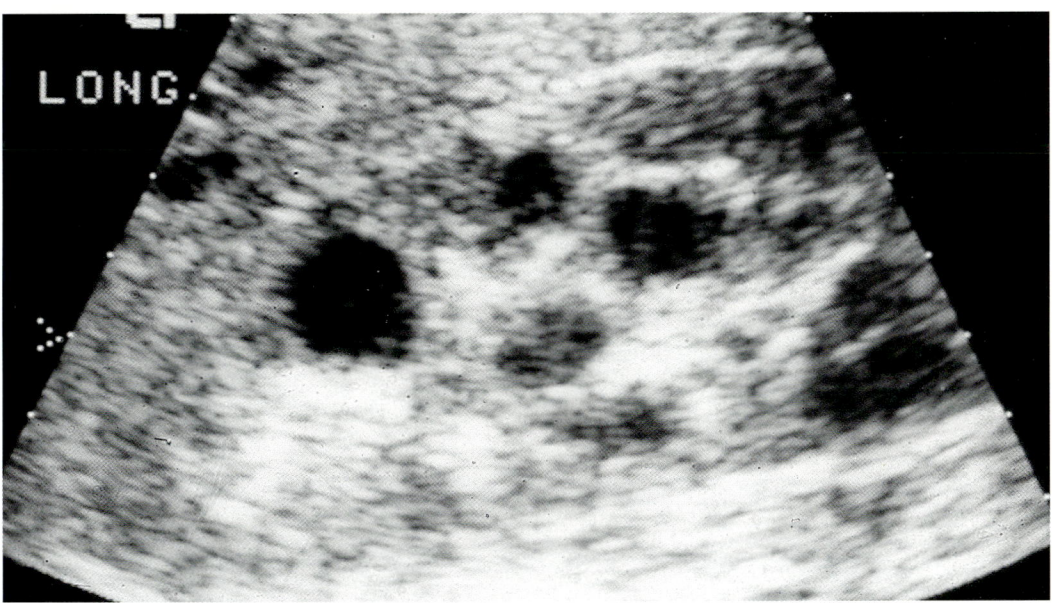

Figure 76 Ultrasonogram (longitudinal view) of a kidney with autosomal-dominant polycystic kidney disease shows an enlarged and cystic right kidney. There is little likelihood of the condition if an ultrasound study in early adulthood is negative. The genetic abnormality associated with the most common form of the disease, designated PKDI, has been localized to the short arm of chromosome 16

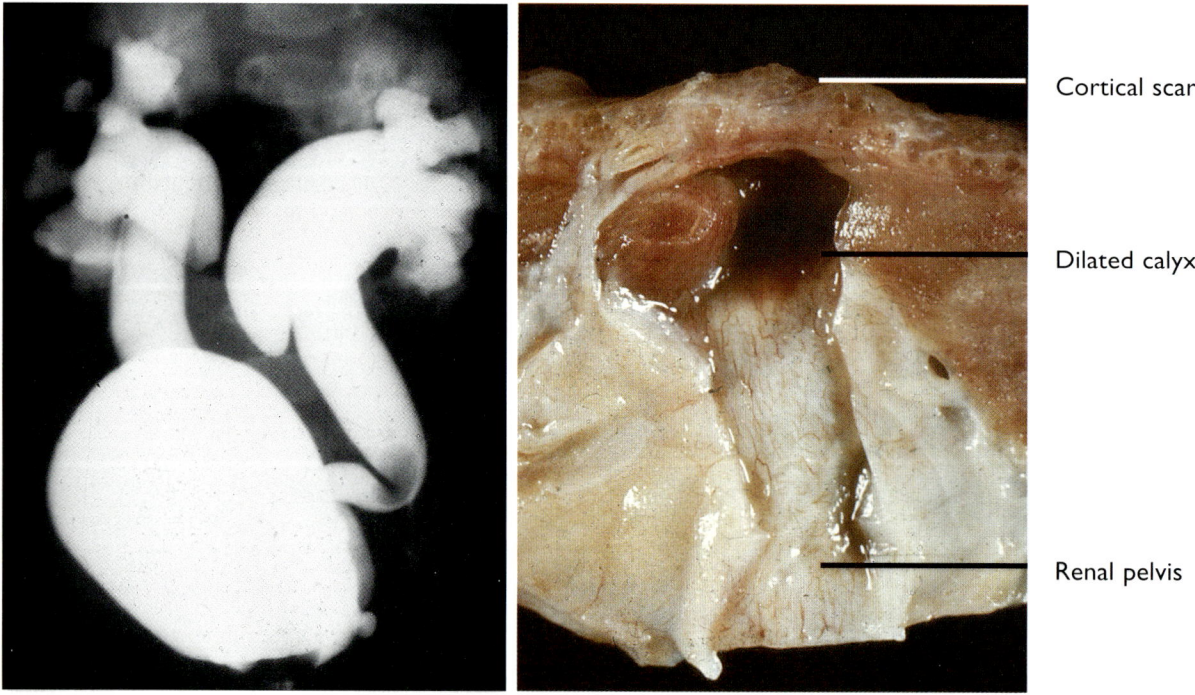

Cortical scar

Dilated calyx

Renal pelvis

Figure 77 Micturating cystogram (left) in an infant with severe vesicoureteric reflux shows intrarenal reflux in the upper poles of the kidneys. In the postmortem specimen (right), one of the dilated calyces shows loss of the overlying parenchyma

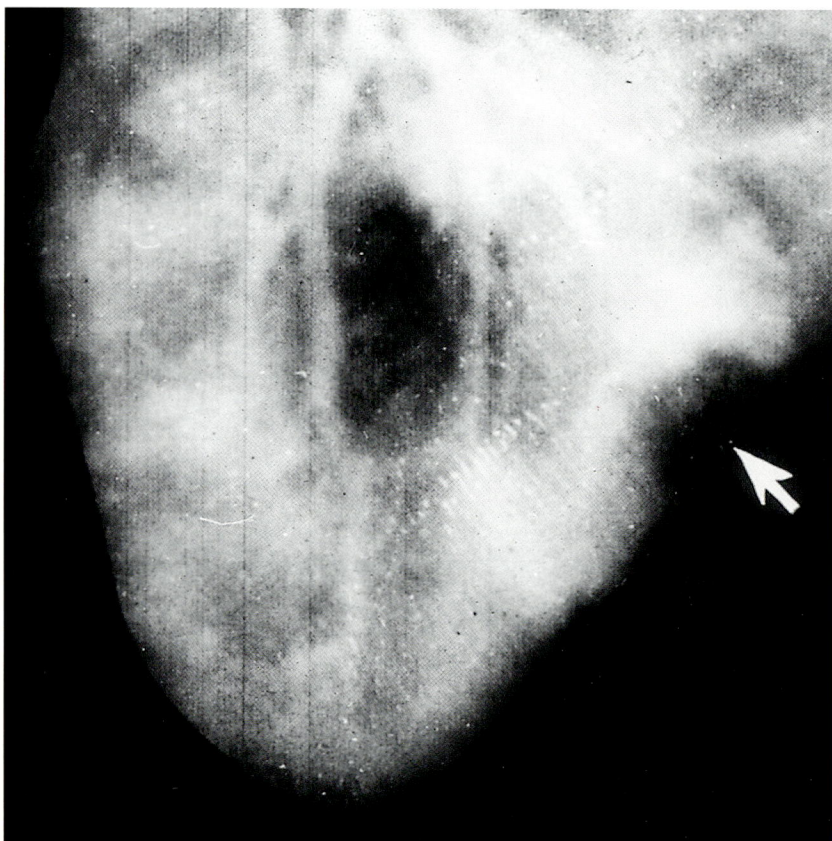

Figure 78 Nephrogram phase of arteriogram of a kidney shows a small defect (arrowed) which proved to be a benign renin-secreting tumor of juxtaglomerular cells. Primary reninism is a rare cause of hypertension and hypokalemia

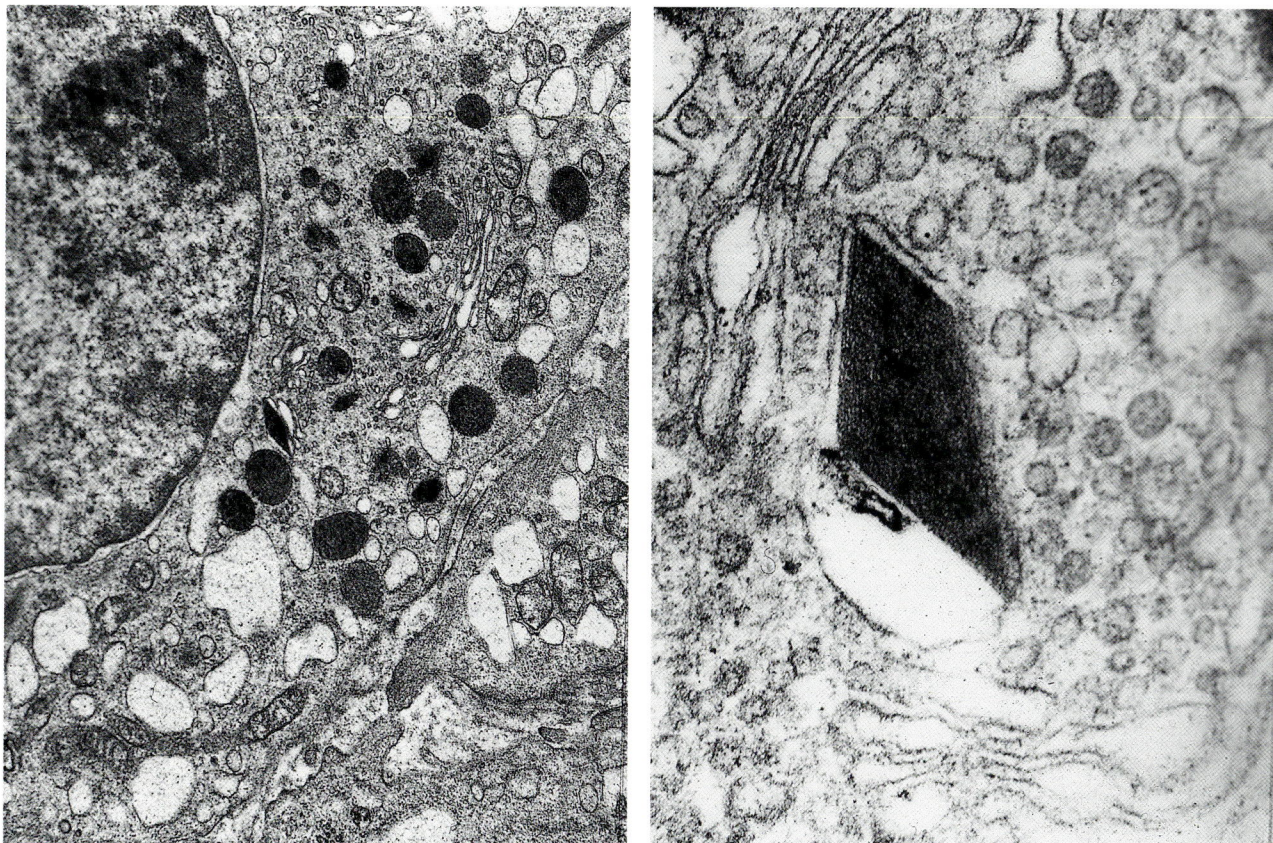

Figure 79 EM of a juxtaglomerular tumor cell shows electron-dense renin granules (left). The rough endoplasmic reticulum is seen as dilated spaces and there is a prominent Golgi apparatus, features of active-phase synthesis and secretion. A typical paracrystalline renin 'protogranule' is lodged in a Golgi apparatus (right)

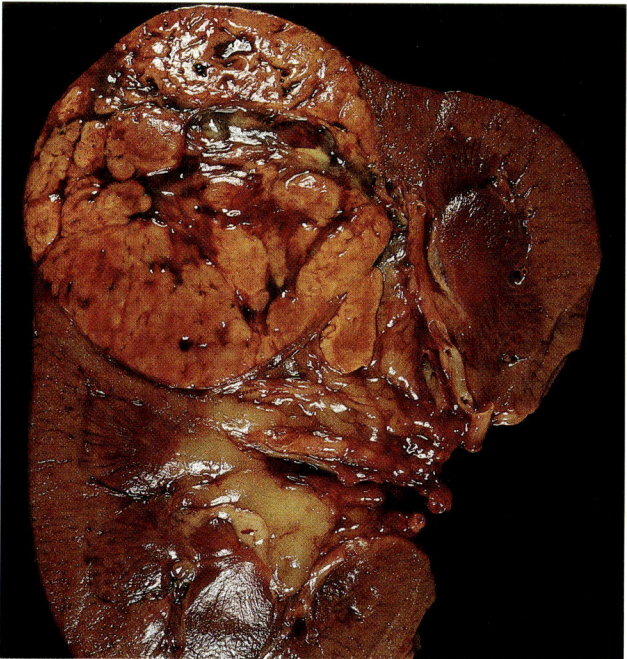

Figure 80 Kidney with a renal cell carcinoma, which may cause hypertension

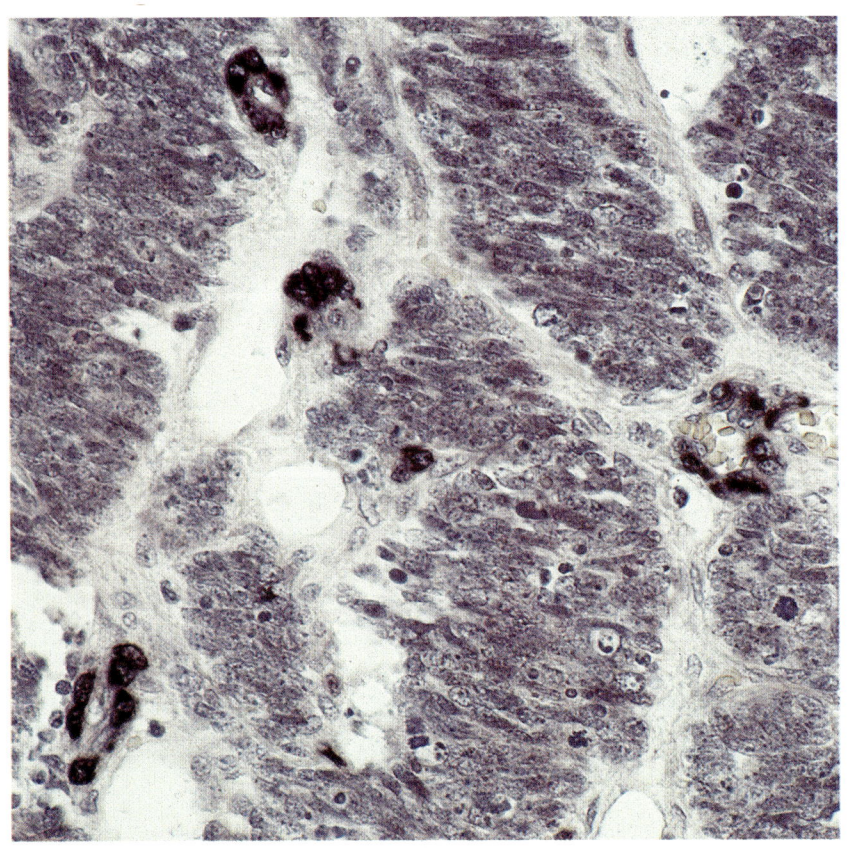

Figure 81 Histology of a blastemic Wilms' tumor showing renin-secreting cells in blood vessels (stained black) by hybridization *in situ* with a probe complementary to human renin mRNA

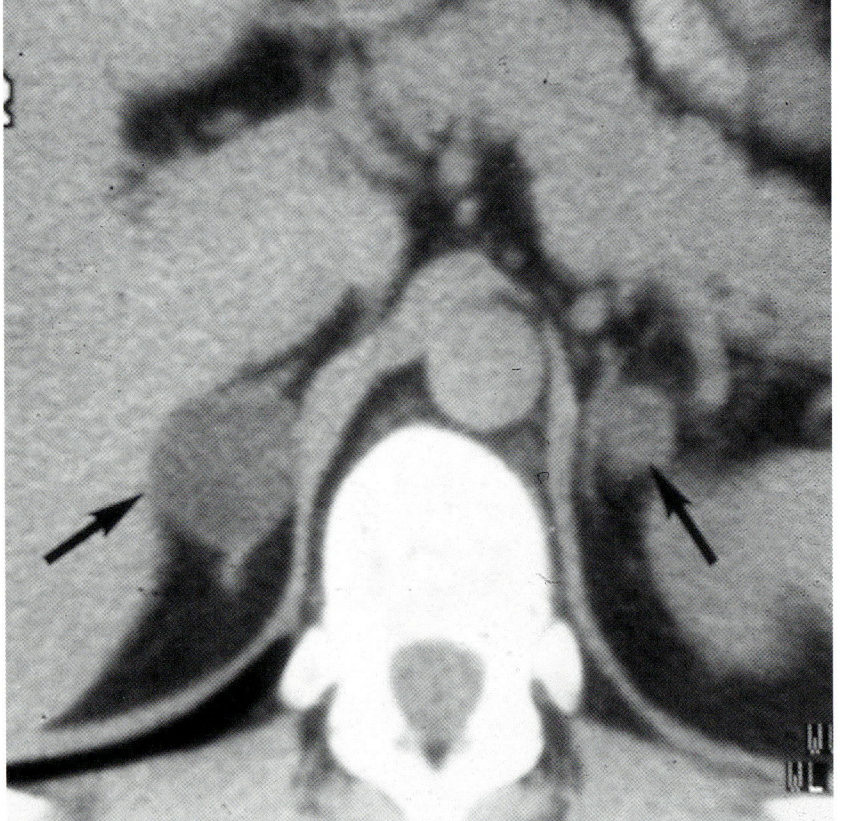

Figure 82 CT of the adrenal glands of a 40-year-old patient with primary aldosteronism showing bilateral tumors, a highly unusual finding as aldosteronomas are virtually always unilateral. In this case, aldosterone secretion was confined to the smaller lesion on the left, demonstrated by aldosterone levels in adrenal venous blood. The larger right-sided lesion had a slightly lower attenuation coefficient and was a non-functioning adenoma

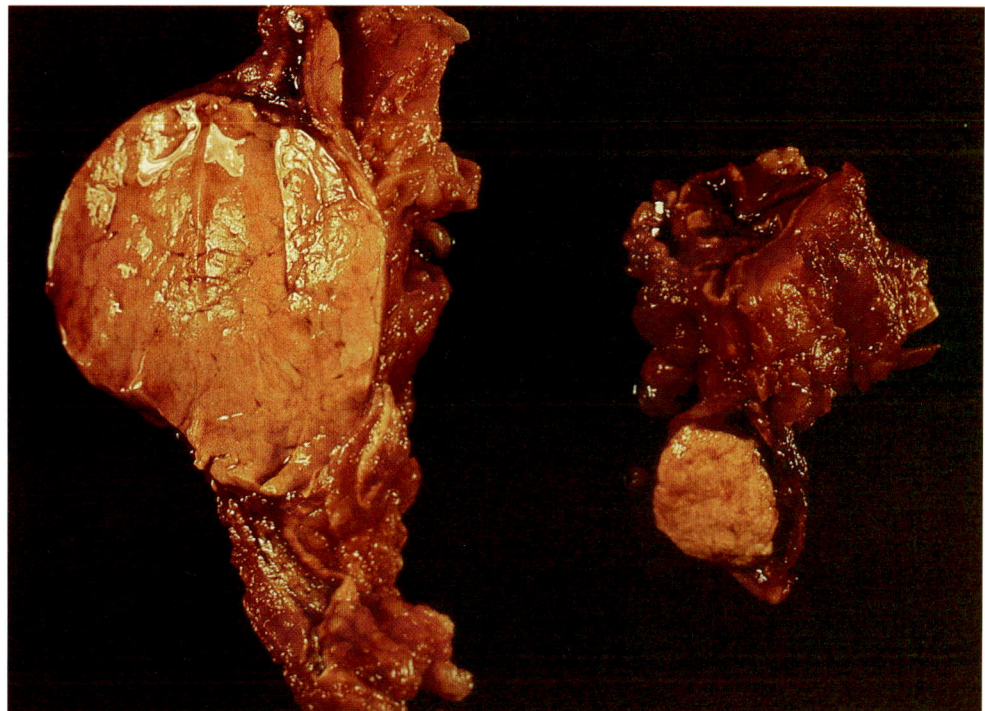

Figure 83 Resected adrenal tumors from the same patient as in Figure 82. Analysis of tumor steroid content demonstrated a high concentration of aldosterone only in the tumor on the left

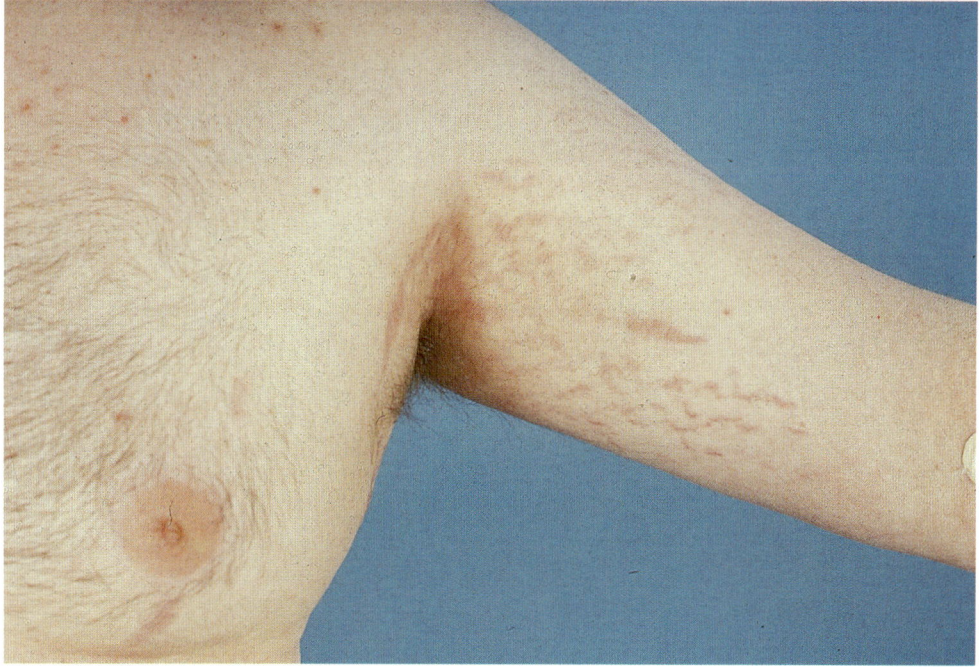

Figure 84 Axillary striae in pituitary-dependent Cushing's disease. The mechanism of the hypertension in Cushing's syndrome has not yet been completely ascertained. Hypokalemia is unusual except in cases with ectopic secretion of adrenocorticotropic hormone (ACTH), most usually from a carcinoid tumor

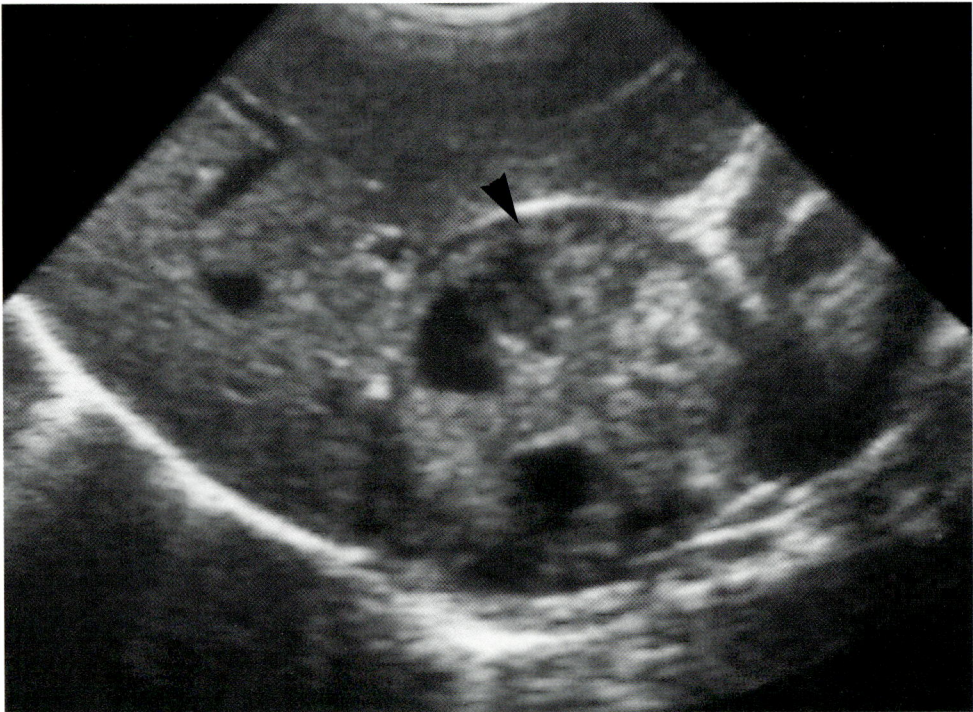

Figure 85 Ultrasonogram of the abdomen showing a large, right adrenal pheochromocytoma (arrowed) containing several fluid-filled areas

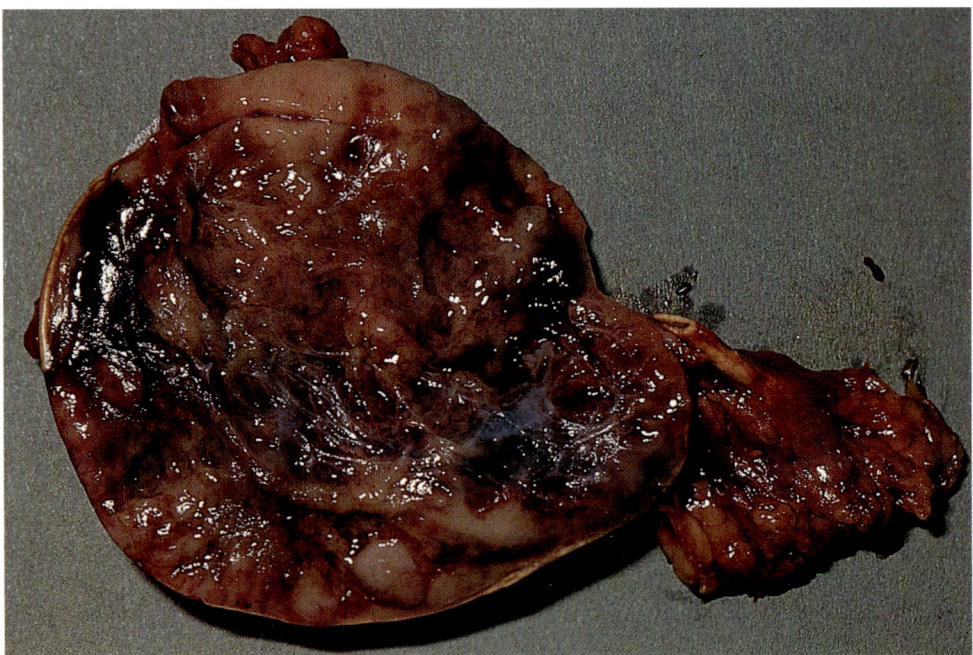

Figure 86 Cut surface of an adrenal pheochromocytoma shows the typical appearance of areas of cystic degeneration and hemorrhage. A vestige of the normal pale-colored gland can just be seen, stretched over the tumor rim. The patient also had neurofibromatosis

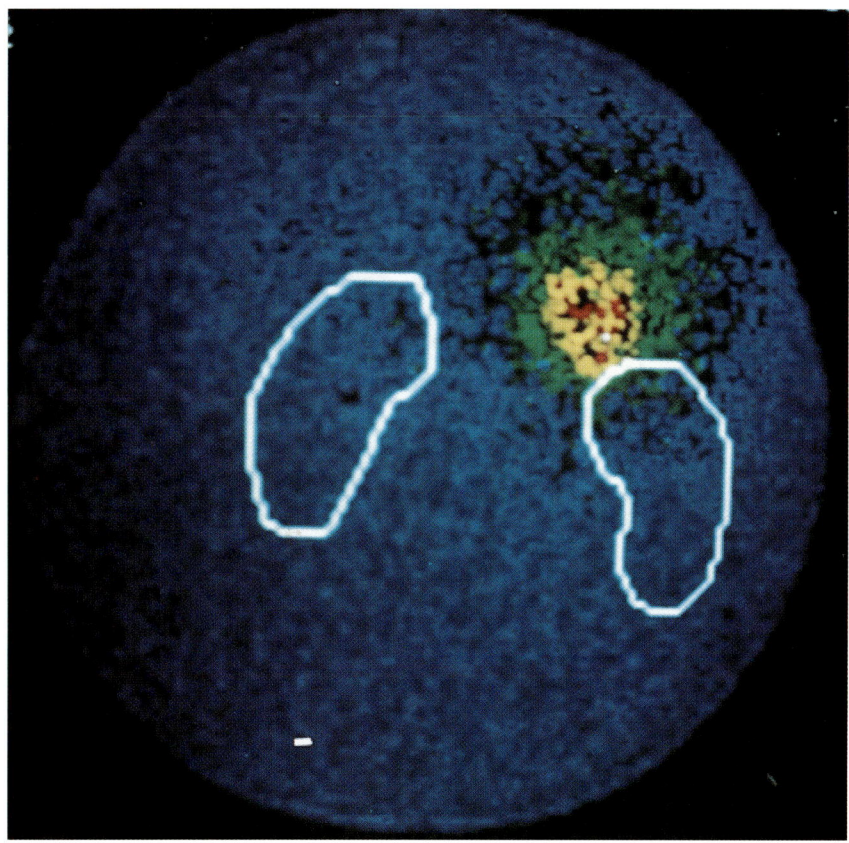

Figure 87 MIBG scintigraphy (posterior view) shows a right adrenal pheochromocytoma. Approximately 80% of these tumors take up radioiodine-labelled meta-iodobenzylguanidine. The modality may be useful in detecting tumor tissue

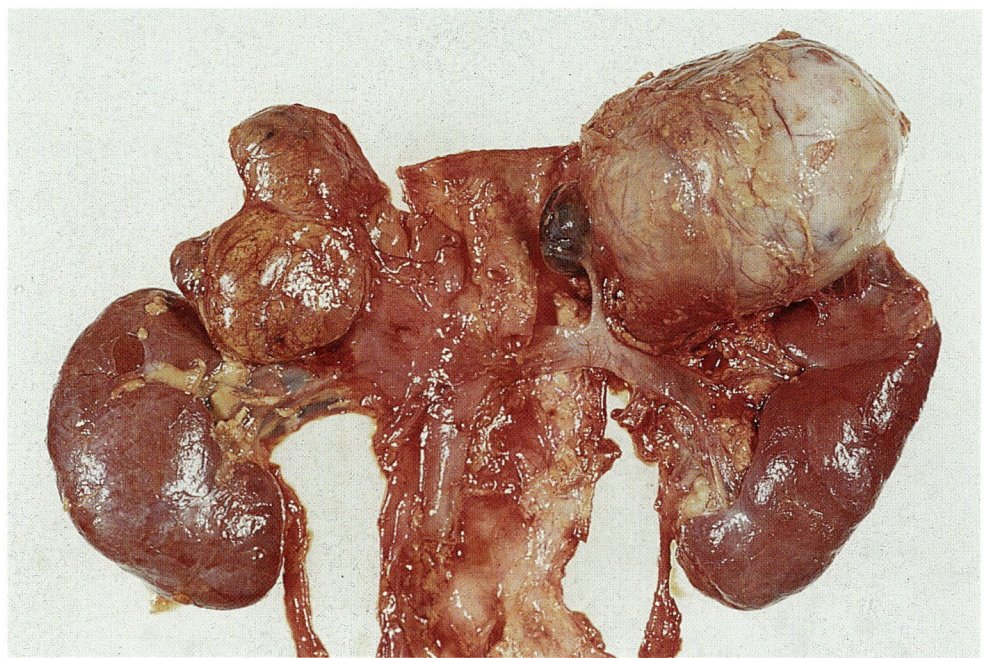

Figure 88 Bilateral adrenal pheochromocytomas due to multiple endocrine neoplasia type IIA, which has a Mendelian-dominant heritability and is caused by a mutation in the RET proto-oncogene. Gene carriers also develop medullary carcinoma of the thyroid

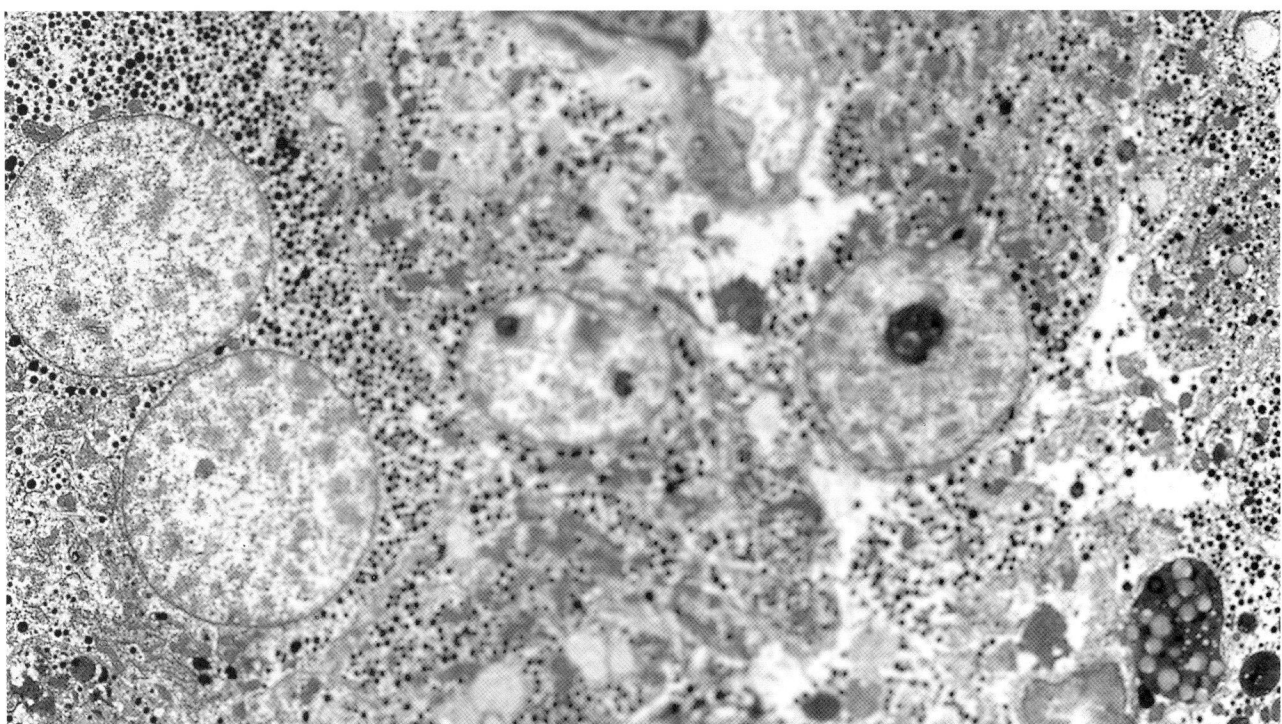

Figure 89 EM of pheochromocytoma showing typical large tumor cells packed with electron-dense catecholamine 'neuroendocrine' granules

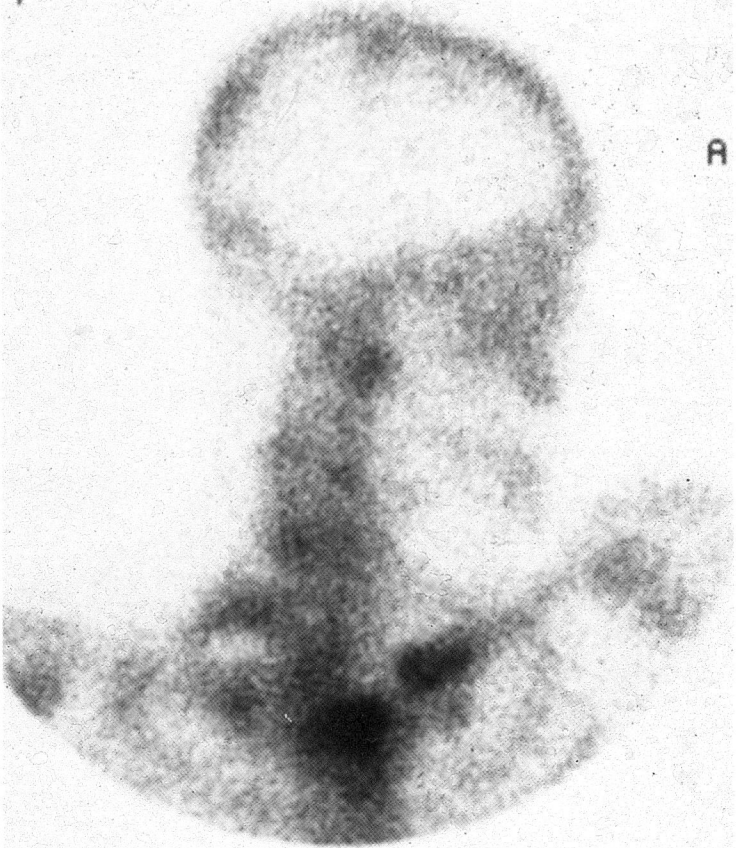

Figure 90 Technetium-labelled methylene diphosphonate bone scan showing secondary deposits of malignant pheochromocytoma in the skull, spine and first left rib

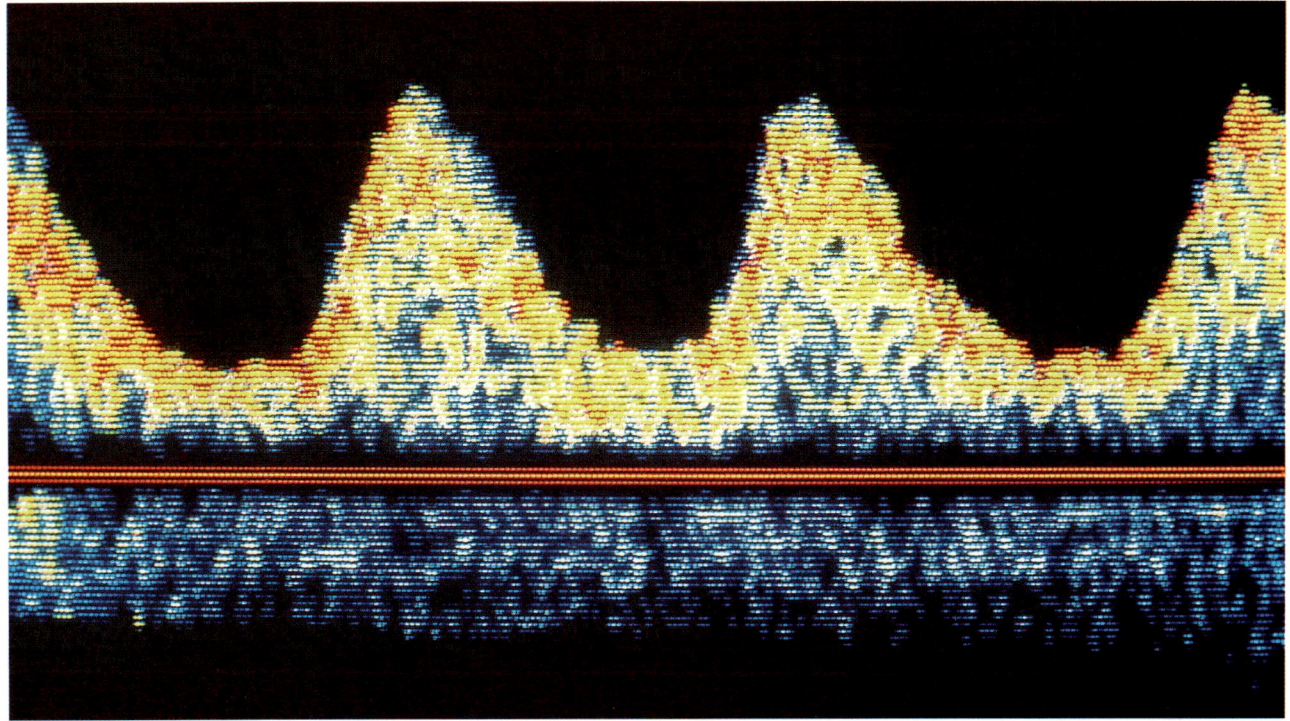

Figure 91 CDI showing normal waveforms in the umbilical artery (above) and vein (below)

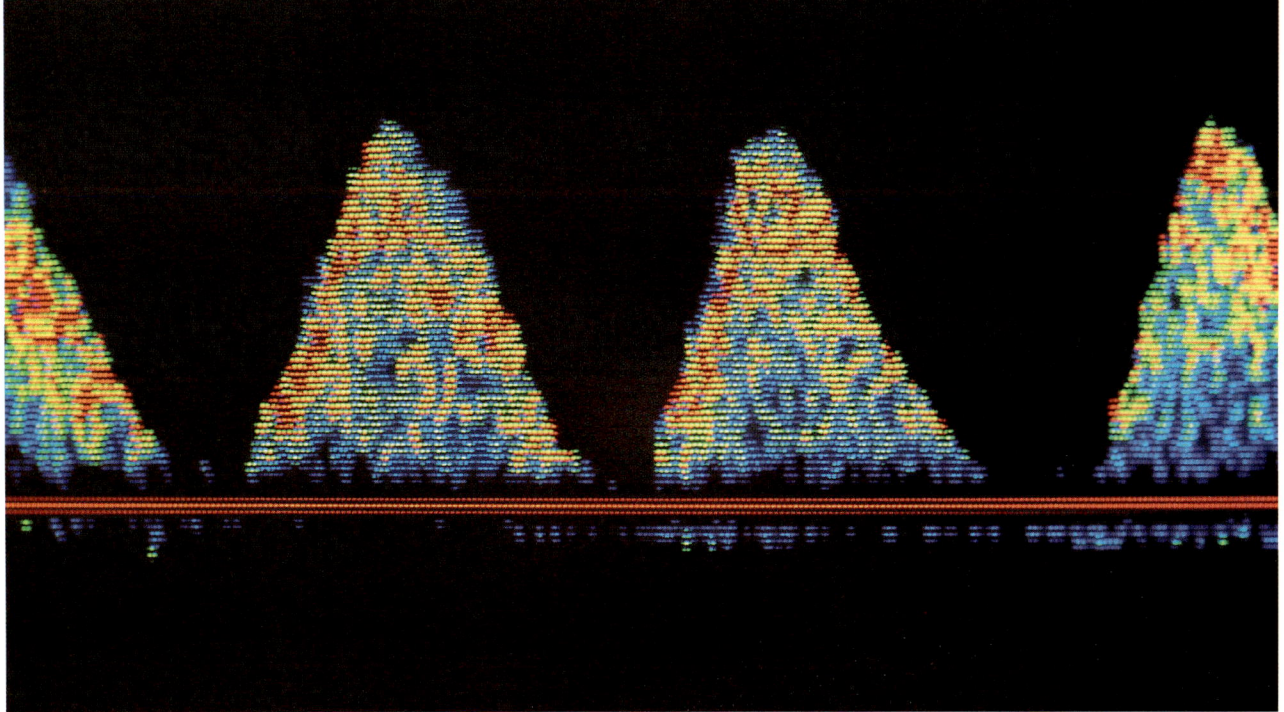

Figure 92 CDI in severe preeclampsia showing abnormal signatures with absent diastolic flow in the umbilical artery (above) and reduced flow in the vein (below). This pattern is associated with marked growth-retardation of the fetus

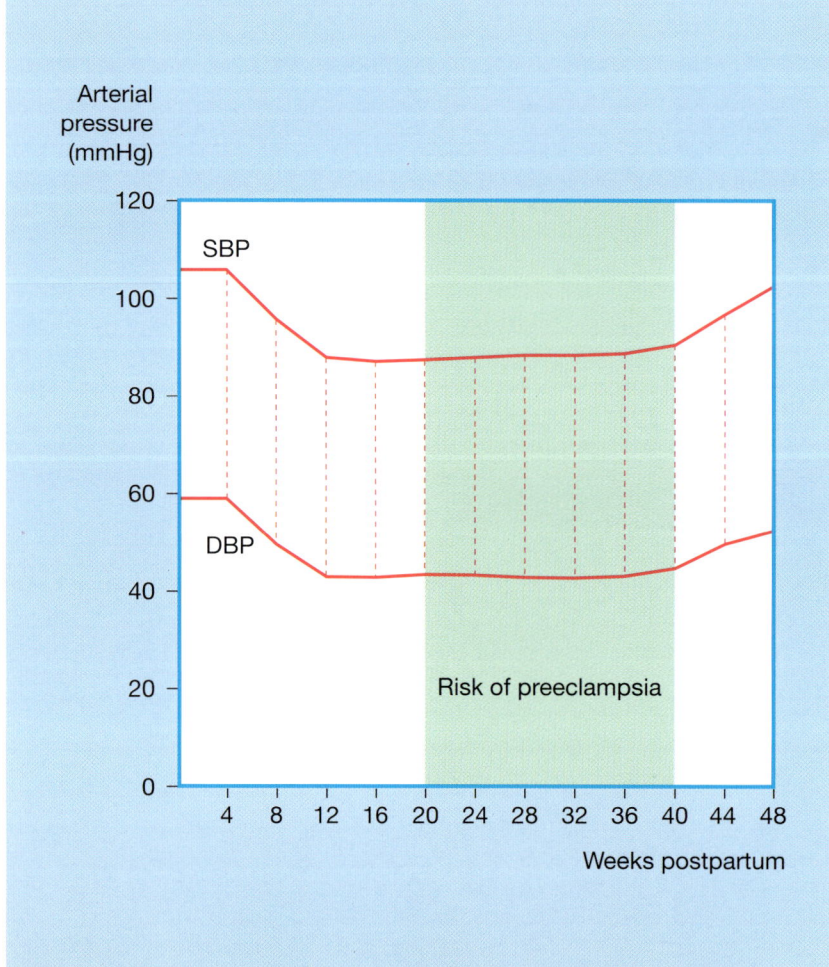

Figure 93 Graph showing the normal pattern of blood pressure in pregnancy. In the last trimester, lower values are obtained in the left lateral position. In the supine position, pressure from the gravid uterus on the inferior vena cava causes narrowing of the pulse pressure due to reflex activation of the sympathetic nervous system. Preeclampsia may develop at any time after week 20 of gestation. Early signs of the condition are hypertension and hyperuricemia followed by proteinuria, thrombocytopenia, hepatic dysfunction and placental impairment

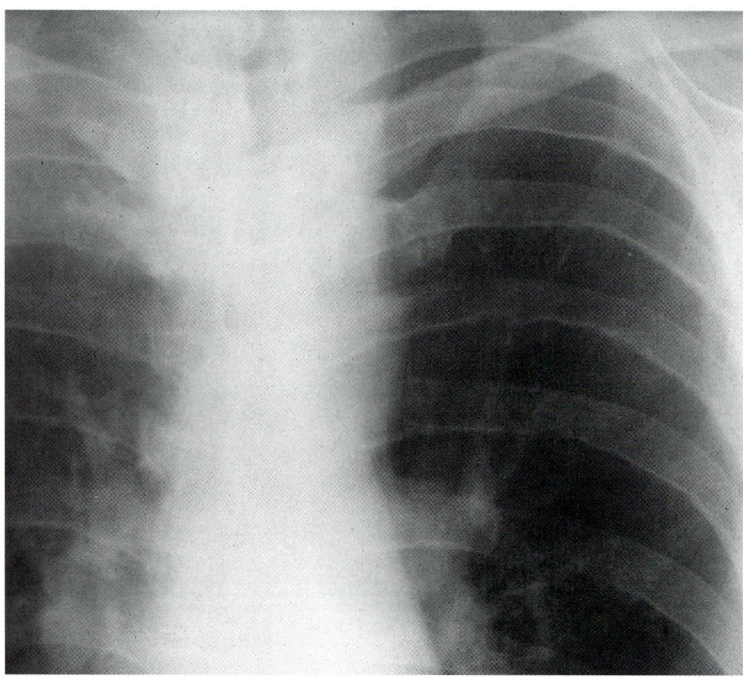

Figure 94 Chest radiograph showing coarctation of the aorta. Enlarged collateral vessels have caused marked notching of the lower margins of the ribs, and the aortic knuckle is reduced. Coarctation is a rare cause of hypertension, but is relatively common in Turner's syndrome (gonadal dysgenesis due to karyotype 45,X)

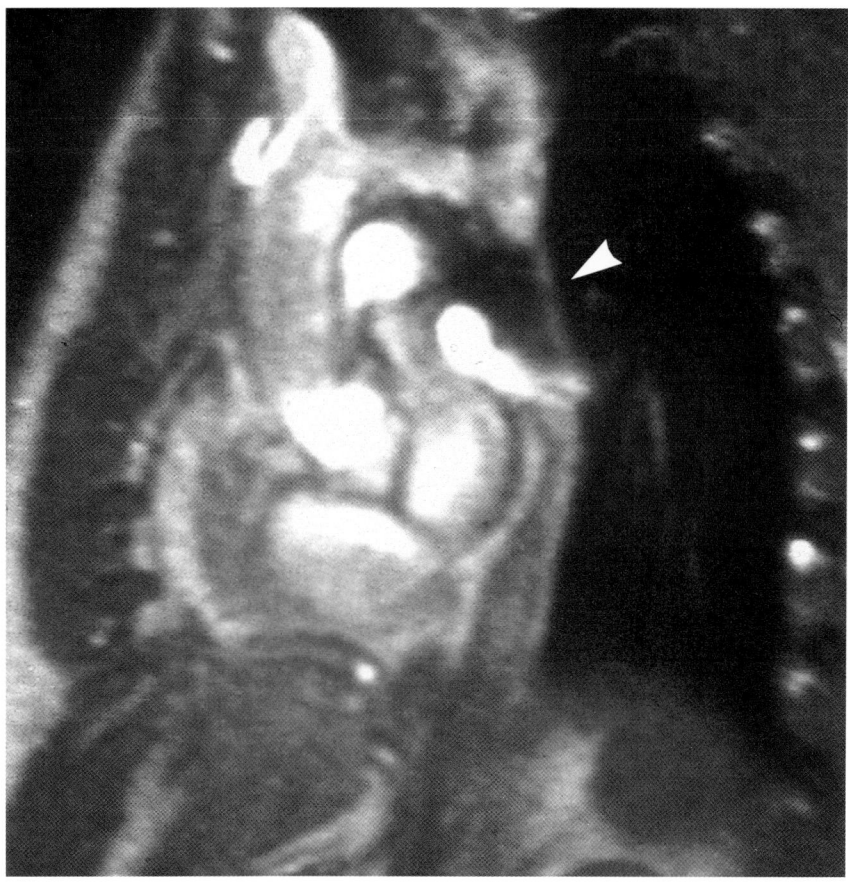

Figure 95 MRI of a 21-year-old patient showing aortic coarctation (arrowed). The patient had symptomless hypertension and impalpable femoral pulses

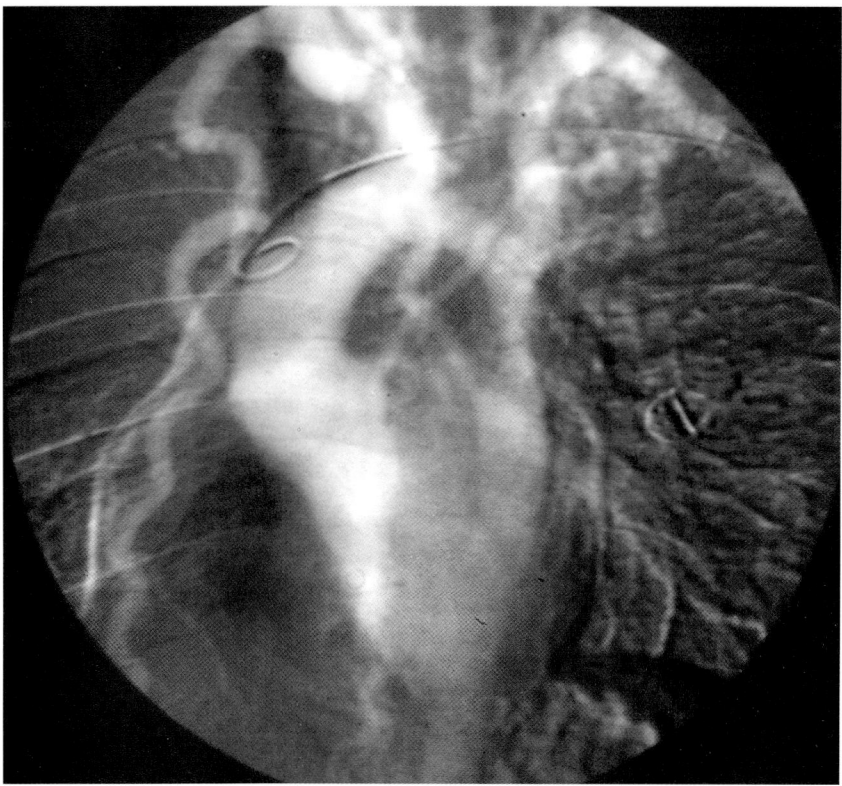

Figure 96 Digital subtraction angiogram of a 14-year-old girl with hypertension and diminished femoral pulses. There is coarctation immediately distal to the left subclavian artery. A greatly enlarged internal mammary artery (on the left) provides collateral flow

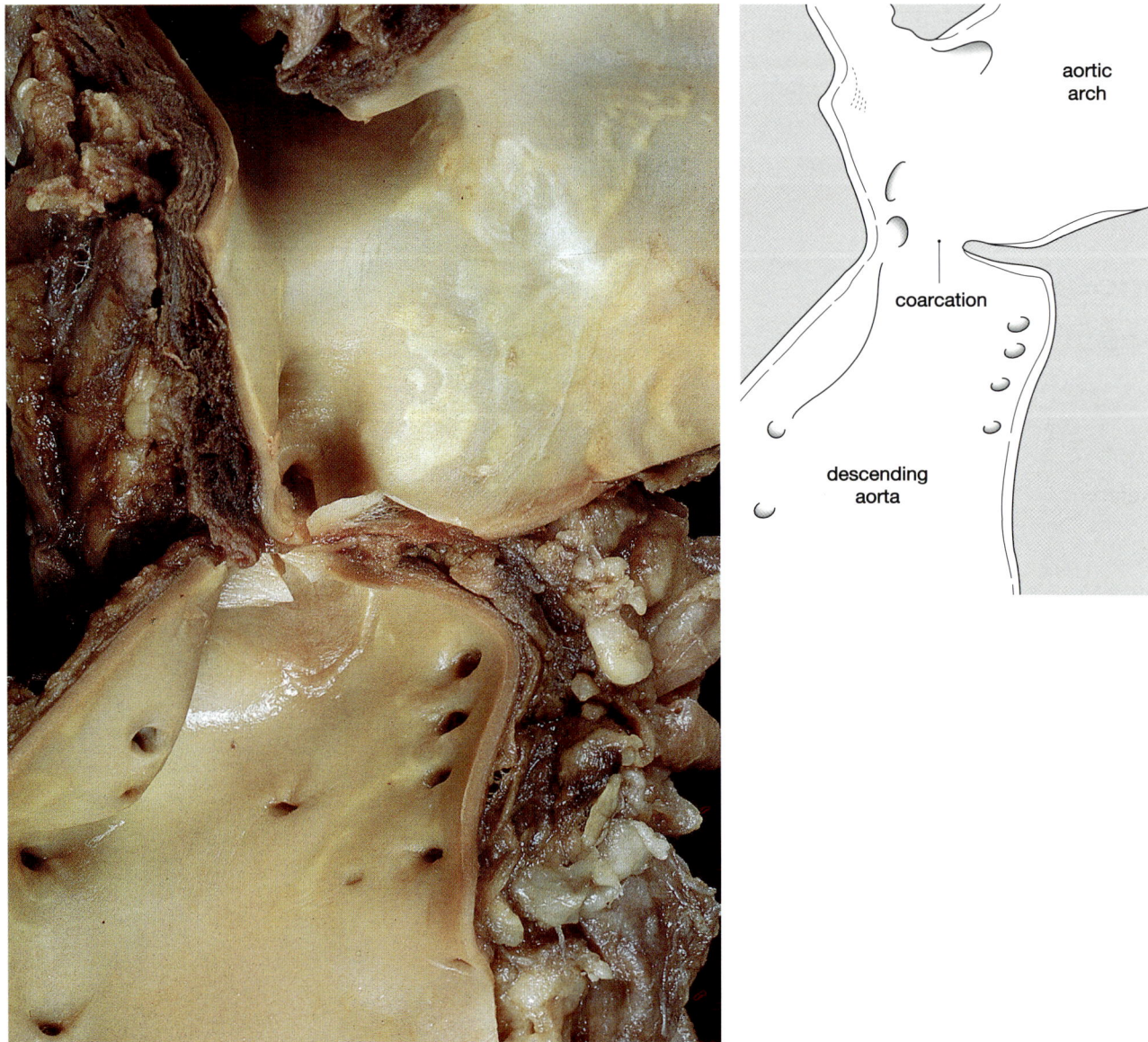

aortic arch

coarcation

descending aorta

Figure 97 Postmortem thoracic aorta showing a tight coarctation just above the origin of the intercostal arteries. Note the presence of early atheroma above, but not below, the coarctation. The 20-year-old patient died due to aortic dissection; marked LVH was also present

Index